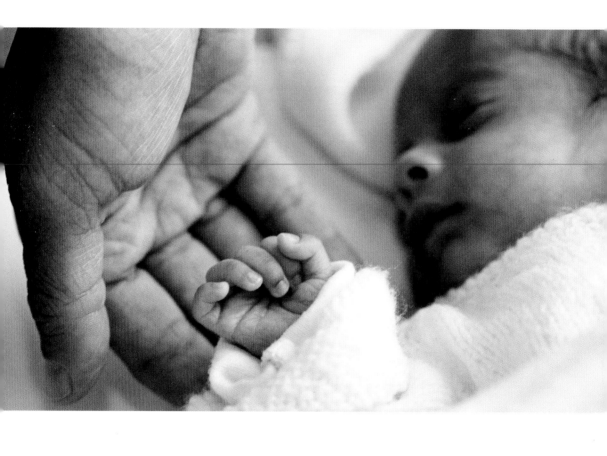

DK your premature baby

looking after your
special care baby
in hospital and at home

Dr Su Laurent & Maya Isaaks

In memory of Felicity Isaaks
21 July 1963 – 22 July 1963

London, New York, Munich, Melbourne, and Delhi

DK UK
Editors Andrea Bagg, Elizabeth Yeates
Designer Saskia Janssen
Senior Production Editor Tony Phipps
Senior Production Controller Seyhan Esen
Creative Technical Support Sonia Charbonnier
New Photography Vanessa Davies
Art Direction for Photography Anne Fisher
Managing Editor Dawn Henderson
Managing Art Editor Christine Keilty
Publisher Peggy Vance

DK INDIA
Editor Kokila Manchanda
Art Editor Divya P R
Managing Art Editor Navidita Thapa
Senior Managing Editor Glenda Fernandes
DTP Designers Anurag Trivedi, Rajdeep Singh
DTP Manager Sunil Sharma

Every effort has been made to ensure that the information in this book is complete and accurate. However, neither the publisher nor the authors are engaged in rendering professional advice or services to the individual reader. The contents of this book are not intended as a substitute for consulting with your healthcare provider. All matters regarding the health of you and your baby require medical supervision. Neither the publisher nor the authors can accept liability or responsibility for any loss or damage allegedly arising from any information or suggestions in this book.

First published in Great Britain in 2012 by
Dorling Kindersley Limited
80 Strand, London WC2R ORL
Penguin Group (UK)

1 2 3 4 5 6 7 8 9 10
001–182741– Oct/2012

A CIP catalogue record for this book is available from the British Library.

ISBN: 978-1-4093-8395-6

Printed and bound in Singapore by TWP

Discover more at www.dk.com

Contents

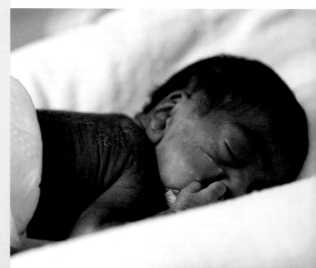

Caring for your baby

Monitoring and treatment

Going home

What the future holds

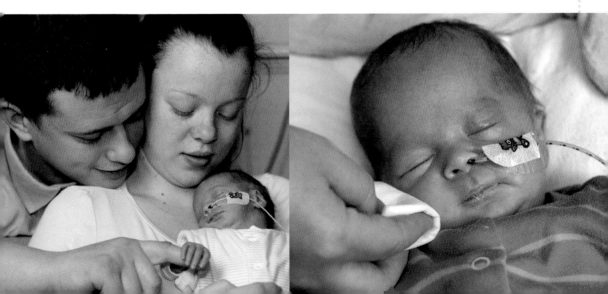

Introduction

When you get the happy news that a baby is on the way, it's natural to hope and indeed expect that everything will go smoothly and your baby will be born at the right time and in perfect health. For some expectant parents, however, things won't go to plan and they will find themselves hearing that their baby is likely to need medical help at or soon after birth.

This book is for you if you have been told that your baby will be born early or with problems that will result in him or her spending time in a neonatal unit. Many parents have told us that they would have liked more information, particularly when they first arrived on the unit.

This book is also for the nurses and doctors who work in a neonatal unit and who would like to understand more about how both parents and babies may feel, and how best to support them through their time on the unit and afterwards.

We are indebted to the many parents who have told us their own stories and allowed us to quote them, and also to the parents who have been happy for us to photograph their precious babies and children. Talking to the nurses and therapists who work in neonatal units has also been a huge part of gathering the information needed to make this a useful and comprehensive book.

You can read this book from beginning to end or you can dip in and out to find more information about specific topics. However you want to use this book, we hope you as parents will feel empowered to support your baby and yourselves during his or her time on the unit, to work in partnership with the medical team, and to play a vital role in your baby's care.

Su Laurent & Maya Isaaks

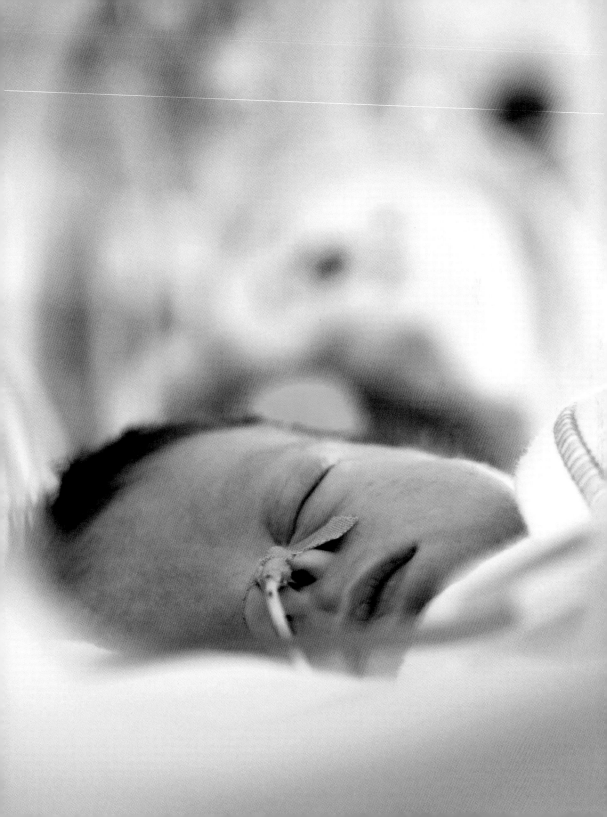

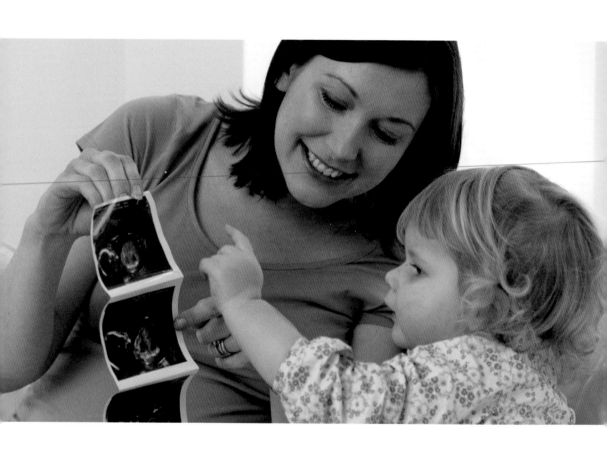

In the beginning

Preparing to meet your new baby is exciting. If she's likely to arrive early, the experienced medical team will do everything to give her the best possible care.

What is prematurity?

Everyone hopes that their pregnancy will go smoothly and that the baby will be born healthy and on time. Sometimes, things don't go to plan and a baby is born early, which means she may need extra care and support.

The normal length of a pregnancy, or gestation, is between 37 and 42 weeks, counted from the first day of your last period. If a baby is born earlier than 37 weeks' gestation, she is considered to be premature. In the UK, around 7.5 per cent of all babies are born prematurely.

If your baby is born too early, her body may not yet be mature enough to cope well with living outside the womb. The kinds of difficulties premature babies can have include breathing, feeding, and coping with infections, so they need to be cared for by a specialist medical team in the hospital's neonatal unit.

As a parent of a premature baby, you may face more uncertainty, complications, and difficult decisions than if your baby had been born at term.

Having a baby earlier than expected can be a very frightening experience, whether you have advance warning or not. Instead of the labour and delivery you imagined and planned for, you are faced with an entirely different scenario, and it's likely to be a very emotional time for you. Rest assured, however, that the expert medical staff taking care of you and your baby before, during, and after the birth will do everything they can to keep you informed and to ensure the best possible outcome. Ask as many questions as you need to, as it's important that you understand what's happening at every stage.

Early arrival Babies born early need help to cope with life outside the womb. This baby is receiving extra oxygen, and milk is being delivered through a tube into her tummy.

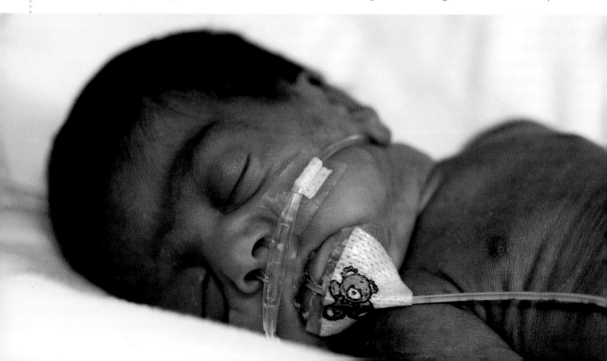

Risks if your baby is born early

With modern technology it is possible for some babies born as early as 23 weeks' gestation to survive, although these babies are more likely to have problems than babies born closer to term.

A baby born at 23 weeks has around a 17 per cent chance of survival, whereas at 25 weeks this rises to 50 per cent. By 28 weeks, a baby born in a hospital has a 90 per cent chance of survival, and this rises with each week she is in the womb. These are just statistics, however, and not a prediction about what will happen to your baby. All babies and experiences are unique.

The womb is the safest environment for your baby. For this reason, when a woman goes into labour very early, the medical team will do everything they can to try to prolong the pregnancy to increase the baby's chance of developing and growing, even if it's just for a couple of days, unless there is a significant risk to the mother or baby.

What's the difference between premature and "small for dates"?

Prematurity simply refers to a baby being born too early. Small-for-dates babies are those who are born smaller than would be expected for a baby of that gestation. Expected sizes throughout gestation are based on centile charts, which plot on a curve the range of weights into which the vast majority of babies fall (see p.117). Generally, a baby who falls below the 2nd centile, meaning that 98 per cent of babies are bigger, is considered small for dates. At term, a small-for-dates baby generally weighs less than 2.5kg (5lb 8oz).

There are various reasons why a premature baby might weigh less than average for her gestational age, and doctors will take these into consideration before concluding that she is small for dates.

A very young or older mum-to-be may be more likely to have a small-for-dates baby, and twins or

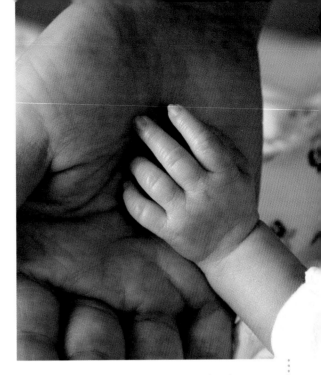

Special care Your premature baby still has a lot of growing to do and will need your comforting presence as well as monitoring and medical support during this time.

more are generally smaller than single babies. Smokers have a higher risk of their babies being smaller than average, and there could also be a medical reason, such as problems with the placenta.

When deciding whether a baby is small for dates, doctors will take the baby's genetic background into account because some ethnic groups naturally have smaller babies. Small parents are also more likely to have a small baby. In these families, a 2.3kg (5lb 2oz) baby who is fit and well wouldn't be considered small for dates, whereas a baby of this weight born to larger parents would be.

Gestational age is much more important in how a baby does than her size at birth. A 600g (1lb 5oz) baby who was born at 26 weeks is small for dates but is likely to do better than a 25-week baby who is 600g (1lb 5oz), even though the 25-weeker is bigger for her gestational age.

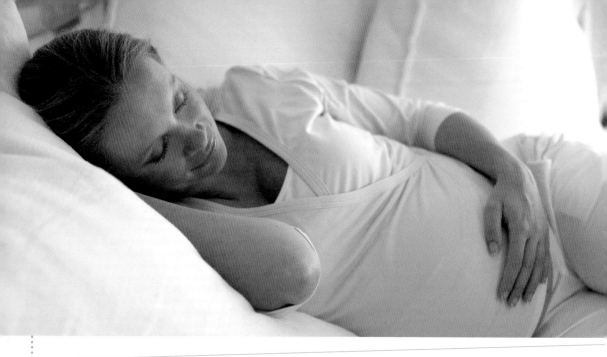

Finding out that your baby may need extra care

If you or your baby has a medical condition, you may have been warned that your baby will be admitted to the neonatal unit when he's born. For many expectant parents, though, the arrival of an early or ill baby comes as a shock.

During pregnancy You may have been told that your baby is likely to be born too early or may need to be admitted to the neonatal unit for another reason. This could be because your unborn baby has been diagnosed with a condition that means he'll need extra help when he's born, or that possibly he'll require an operation.

Whatever the reason, hearing that your baby will not be coming home with you soon after birth is understandably very worrying, and it's helpful to find out as much as you can about what is likely to happen at birth and immediately afterwards. The more you understand about what may happen

to your baby, the better you will be able to cope with this difficult situation.

If there is time before the birth, it's a good idea to visit the unit and talk to the staff about what to expect. A doctor or nurse can show you round and give you an idea of what your baby may look like and how small he may be. You can see the equipment he may need and ask about how long he is likely to stay in the unit. It will probably look very scary initially, but it's reassuring to prepare yourself and feel that your baby will be in safe hands.

If you are unable to visit the unit, one of the doctors who will be looking after your baby should

Look after yourself If you know your baby may be born early, try to prepare by eating well and resting as much as possible. Get help with older children if you can.

be able to come and see you on the labour ward and tell you what to expect. She will aim to be as reassuring as possible but will also be honest to help you think of questions to ask and to help you remember what was said. Often, there won't be a straightforward answer to your question as the situation usually becomes clearer once a baby has been born. For some lucky parents, the anxiety about a predicted premature delivery proves unfounded and the baby arrives at the right time.

> "We knew that he was going to be early but you don't understand what's to come in terms of the depth of care, how delicate it is, and how traumatic it can be."
>
> *Ross, dad to Freddie*

about your baby's chances if he is likely to be born extremely early or has a condition that means he will not live. It's always best to have this conversation with your partner present. If it's not possible for your partner to be there, you might want to have a friend or family member with you

At delivery Sometimes, despite a straightforward pregnancy, there are problems during labour or you unexpectedly go into labour early. Suddenly you find yourself thrown into turmoil as the obstetric team monitor your contractions and check the baby's heartbeat for

MY STORY
Cher says...

"I was 31 weeks and I just knew something wasn't right, so I phoned the hospital. My blood pressure was a bit high and I'd had pre-eclampsia with my first son so they told me to come in.

Once my blood pressure had settled they said 'We'll just check the baby'. His heart rate was so high they thought the monitor had broken. A really experienced midwife came in and after looking at the monitor asked how long had it been showing those readings. I said, 'on and off', and within seconds a doctor came flying in – my baby's heart rate was 280 and it was meant to be 160. Then they were telling me to take my earrings out. They delivered my baby straight away by Caesarean section, and I was allowed to see him briefly before they took him to special care and ventilated him. From there it was an emotional roller coaster, because it took them a while to realize it was a condition called supraventricular tachycardia (SVT), which means his heart can go double the rate it's meant to be in the blink of an eye. Not only were they trying to manage his heart, they were also trying to manage his prematurity. No end of times, I thought they were going to tell me he was dead because I couldn't understand how he could carry on living with his heart rate going that fast when he was so small. For a premature baby at 31 weeks he was 1.8kg (4lb), which was quite a good weight, so we had that on our side. "

Cher, mum to Xavier

signs of distress. There is no time to prepare yourselves for this traumatic change of plan, but you can trust that the staff surrounding you are doing everything they can for you and your baby.

In a situation where there are signs of fetal distress, such as unusual variations in the baby's heartbeat, you may be told that an emergency

Whether you're having a natural birth or a Caesarean section, the neonatal team will do their best to keep you fully informed throughout and, if possible, will show you your baby before taking him to the neonatal unit.

A baby may need to be resuscitated because he has suffered from a lack of oxygen during labour

> " I didn't see her when she was born. I had placental abruption and they said, 'We've got to get her out now.' She was in a bad way, and it was really touch and go. "
>
> *Carolyn, mum to Evie*

Caesarean section is necessary. This can be done under epidural or spinal anaesthesia if there is time or if you already have an epidural in place. However, if the neonatal team have great concern about your baby's well-being, you will be advised to have a general anaesthetic as it is faster.

or delivery, or because he has inhaled meconium, the tarry poo that a baby sometimes passes before delivery because he is in distress. Resuscitation can involve giving extra oxygen, suction of the mouth and nose, and gentle stimulation, which may consist of gently rubbing the baby. Sometimes, a baby

Am I in labour?

If you have any of the following signs that labour may be starting or is likely to start before 37 weeks of pregnancy, it's important to seek medical advice straight away:

• A show (pink or brown mucus discharge). During pregnancy your cervix is blocked by a plug of mucus that prevents bacteria reaching your baby. If you notice a pink or brown jelly-like discharge, this may be the mucus plug coming away and can be a sign that labour may start soon.

• Your waters breaking (rupture of the amniotic membranes surrounding your baby). You may notice a slow trickle of liquid – and may wonder whether you've wet yourself – or you may

experience a gush of fluid. Either way, you should always check with your midwife or doctor if you think the amniotic sac has ruptured.

• Regular contractions, which may feel like period pains to start with and are likely to become stronger and more frequent.

You should also seek urgent medical advice if you experience any of the signs listed below. They may not mean you are in labour, but may indicate there is a problem and should be checked immediately.

• Lower abdominal pain
• Vaginal bleeding
• Lower back pain
• A bad headache or visual disturbances
• Reduced fetal movements.

who has been in a lot of distress before or during delivery may not breathe at all at birth and will require more active help to start breathing (see Ventilator, p.30)

Sometimes a baby is born with a problem, such as a heart defect, that has not been diagnosed during pregnancy and for which treatment will be needed on the neonatal unit.

On the postnatal ward
Occasionally everything appears to be going very well. The baby is born at or near term with a good Apgar score (see p.20) and the midwife is happy that the baby is healthy. But then a problem arises. This may be something specific you notice yourself, such as your baby seeming irritable, floppy, or blue, or you may just feel that something is not right. Or it may be that the midwife or doctor spots a possible problem, for example, features suggestive of a syndrome such as Down's. They should share their concerns with you in a clear and honest way and explain what will happen next. The medical team should allow you to ask any questions and make sure you feel that your baby is in safe hands.

Sometimes your baby may need to be transferred to the neonatal unit for tests and observation for a short time but can then be treated and monitored on the postnatal ward.

On other occasions, your baby will need to be admitted to the neonatal unit for close monitoring and detailed investigations in order to work out the diagnosis and plan the appropriate treatment. In some ways this is particularly hard as you have had no time to prepare yourselves for this sudden change of plan, and have already told your friends and family that all is well with your baby.

Whatever the situation, it will help you to cope with the days and weeks ahead if you understand what is happening and make sure that you remain fully informed throughout.

MY STORY
Claudia says...

"I was pregnant with identical twins, and at my 20-week scan everything was fine. At 23 weeks my waters broke.

They didn't hold out much hope for the babies, but I had steroid injections to develop their lungs. I went into labour the next morning and I delivered naturally. My son Alfie was stillborn and Chase was not in a good way. Chase was taken straight away to intensive care. He was monitored up and given lots of different medications and blood tests. He was tiny, he was very, very sick, and it was very desperate for a long time.

It was as if it had happened to someone else. I didn't expect to keep either of them, so I'm lucky I've got Chase."

Claudia, mum to Chase

Welcome to the world Even when a baby is born very early, dad may still be able to cut the umbilical cord and will be able to stay close by while he's checked over.

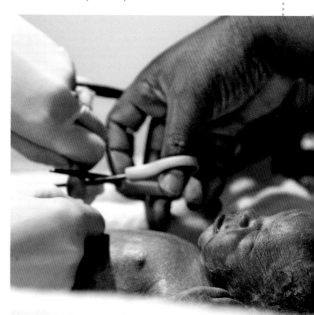

Why has this happened to my baby?

This is one of the first questions parents are likely to ask. Often doctors don't know why a baby is born early, but there is very rarely anything you could have done to avoid it, so try not to feel guilty – it's not your fault.

Mums often feel guilty and worried that they may have done something during pregnancy to cause their baby's prematurity or other problems, or that somehow their body has let their baby down. You might think: "What did I do wrong?", "Why did my baby get this infection?", "Was it because I carried on exercising?" but often there are no answers and there is usually nothing you could have done to change the outcome for your baby. As hard as it may be to believe, sometimes these things just happen,

> **"** I was certain it was something I'd done, that I'd brought it on myself, that it was down to me. I needed someone to tell me it wasn't my fault. **"**
>
> *Carolyn, mum to Evie*

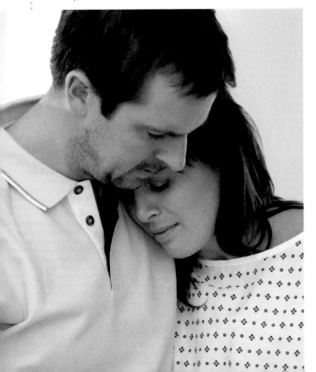

Feeling guilty It's perfectly normal to wonder why your baby has been born early, but there is usually no explanation that doctors can find.

but many mums of premature or ill babies find it very hard to let go of feeling responsible.

If you're struggling with these feelings, try to remember that what has happened to your baby is not your fault. This is an overwhelming and challenging time for parents. It's important for dads to be supportive, and to reassure their partner that she is not to blame for what's happened.

Doctors often don't know why babies are born prematurely. In fact, they don't even completely understand what makes a woman go into labour, whether at term or otherwise. Even when looking at whether hormone changes trigger labour to start, it is unclear why these changes happen. A woman can have a premature baby in one pregnancy and then go on to have a baby who is born at term. However, if you have had a premature baby, the chance of having another one is increased. Studies show that the recurrence rate for mothers of premature babies is between 20 per cent and 50 per cent, but every case is different.

Occasionally, a pregnant woman will suffer some form of physical trauma, such as a car accident or being a victim of violence, and in these cases the physical trauma might be responsible for her baby's prematurity – although it is rare to know for sure. Usually, though, everything seems fine, and then suddenly a woman will go into a premature labour.

Possible causes of prematurity

In 40 per cent of cases of premature birth, the cause is unknown. In the remaining 60 per cent, there are a number of possible causes, listed below. Some of these may trigger an early labour, while others require your baby to be delivered early for the sake of your or your baby's health.

- Illness in the mother, such as high blood pressure or diabetes, and certain infections.
- Expecting twins or more – about half of twins, and nearly 90 per cent of triplets – are born early.
- Smoking during pregnancy.
- Placental abruption, in which the placenta comes away from the wall of the womb, reducing the blood and oxygen supply to the baby.
- Pre-eclampsia, a condition occurring during pregnancy in which the mother develops high blood pressure accompanied by protein in the urine; it can reduce the blood flow to the baby and is potentially dangerous for the mother.
- Cervical incompetence, in which the cervix is not strong enough to stay tightly closed as the baby grows bigger and heavier; even a stitch inserted during pregnancy is not always enough to prevent the baby coming early.
- Problems with the baby, such as too much or too little amniotic fluid, an infection, or when a baby has died.

It is important to reiterate that, in many cases, the cause of premature birth is not known and there was either little or nothing you could have done to prevent it occurring.

TWINS AND TRIPLETS
Twin-to-twin transfusion

Twin-to-twin transfusion is a rare condition occurring only in identical twins in which blood passes from one twin to the other when in the womb. One baby ends up with too much blood while the other has too little, which can cause problems, and the babies may have to be delivered early.

At birth, the twin who has donated blood is often smaller and is pale and anaemic, while the twin who received too much blood is larger, with increased blood pressure. Treatment can include a blood transfusion for the anaemic twin and removal of blood from the twin with too much blood. If the problem is detected before birth, some hospitals may be able to offer laser treatment to block the flow of blood from one baby to the other.

Identical twins Only identical twins who share a placenta are at risk of twin-to-twin transfusion, but even in these babies the condition is rare.

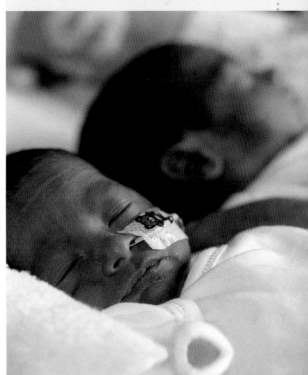

What will my baby look like?

Your premature baby will look quite different from a baby born at term. As well as being small, he won't have much body fat and, depending on how early he is, he may be very floppy, with thin skin and fine body hair.

Parents often worry about what their premature baby will look like, but however early they arrive, all babies will be fully formed and have all their bits! If your baby is born early, how he looks will depend on what gestation he is. Doctors will look at different characteristics in a baby to assess his stage of development, including:

Eyes At 25 weeks, your baby's eyelids may be open, but they could still be fused closed. By 30 weeks, though, his eyes will be wide open.

> " Max came out in a sac, like Erin. I knew exactly what he'd look like: a little skinned chicken. He had these tiny arms and tiny legs. "
>
> *Dana, mum to Erin and Max*

Creases If your baby is born at 25 weeks, you'll notice that her hands and feet are smooth. If she's born at 35 weeks, she will have lots more creases.

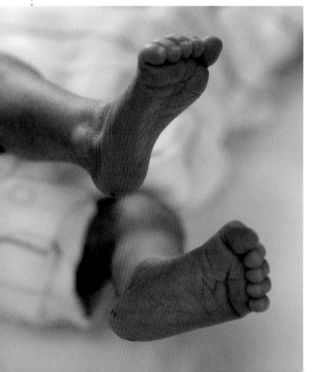

Ears A baby's ear cartilage doesn't develop until week 35, giving the ears a firm appearance. Until then, their ears are very soft and can fold over.

Creases in the hands and feet A 25-week baby's hands and feet will be smooth at birth, a 30-weeker's will have a few little creases on them, and those of a 35-week baby will have lots more.

Nipples A 25-week baby will have immature-looking nipples that are very flat. A 35-week baby will have little nipples that look much more like a normal-term baby's, and a 30-weeker's nipples will be somewhere in between.

Genitals In a little boy at 25 weeks, the testes can't be felt and he will have a rather small and smooth-looking scrotum, whereas at 30 weeks the testes probably can be felt, and at 35 weeks they can certainly be felt. In a baby girl at 25 weeks, the labia majora (outer genital folds) will not cover the labia minora (inner folds), at 30 weeks they will probably almost cover them, and at 35 weeks they will completely cover them.

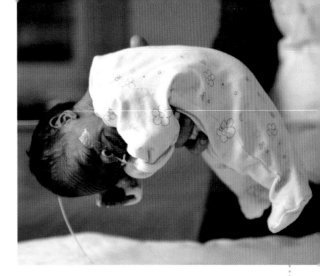

Skin Doctors will look at skin thickness, as the earlier a baby is born, the thinner, more fragile, and more gelatinous his skin will be.

Veins Because a very premature baby will have thin skin, the blood vessels will show more clearly, so the closer to term your baby is born, the less you'll be able to see of his veins.

Lanugo This is hair that grows on your baby's body, particularly his back, while he's in the womb. Usually it has disappeared by the time a baby has reached term. Extremely premature babies may not yet have lanugo, but many premature babies can be rather hairy.

Vernix Premature babies often have very little vernix – the white, greasy substance that protects the baby's skin while he is in the womb.

Flexibility The medical team will look at how bendy a baby is; the more premature the baby, the more flexible he will be. There are different signs doctors can look for, such as how far across his body a baby's arm will bend (called the "scarf sign") and how close his heel can get to his ear.

Floppiness If a 25-week baby is held face down on your hand, his whole body will droop, whereas by 35 weeks he may make an effort to hold up his arms and legs.

Reflexes Babies are born with primitive reflexes, involuntary responses that gradually disappear over the first few months of life. These reflexes are nature's way of helping baby mammals to survive, although some are not important to human babies.

Primitive reflexes include the grasp, or palmar, reflex, in which if you put your finger in a baby's palm, his fingers will instinctively grip one of your fingers; the startle, or Moro, reflex, in which a baby will thrust out his arms if his head or neck is unsupported; and the stepping reflex, in which your baby will place one foot in front of the other as you support his weight. These reflexes indicate that your

Floppy babies If a very premature baby is held face down, her whole body will droop as she is not yet mature enough to try to hold up her head or limbs.

baby's nervous system is in good working order. All these reflexes are usually present by 30 weeks' gestation, and, remarkably, some very premature babies of 25 weeks' gestation are born with some of them, such as the grasp and startle reflexes. At 25 weeks, your baby won't yet have a sucking reflex, so he won't be put to the breast to feed. At 35 weeks, though, or even a few weeks earlier, it's worth putting him to the breast just for the feeling and smell, even if he's not yet ready to breastfeed.

Dubowitz score Within the first 24 hours of a baby being born prematurely, some doctors use a list of physical and neurological criteria called the Dubowitz score to assess his developmental stage. These criteria are useful for working out the gestational age of a baby if there is any uncertainty about this. Determining the Dubowitz score includes checking all the characteristics listed opposite. So if you see a doctor moving your premature baby's foot to his ear or pulling him up by the arms to see how much his head goes back, he or she may be doing this assessment. Don't worry – these checks won't hurt your baby at all.

What happens when a baby is born early?

When a premature baby is about to arrive, the medical team will be standing by with all the equipment they need to check her over straight away and give her any medical help she needs.

If your baby is premature or is thought likely to have problems, there will generally be one or two paediatricians and a neonatal nurse on hand. If you are having more than one baby, there will be more staff. A special cot known as a resuscitaire, which has a heater, oxygen, suction, and monitoring equipment, will be ready to use.

Strange as it may sound, your premature baby might be delivered into a plastic bag to keep her warm as she's carried over to the resuscitaire. She

and 2, which are then added together to give an Apgar score, with 10 the highest score. Many babies have a low score at one minute, but a good score at five.

First breaths If the baby is not making any obvious breaths and needs some help with breathing, she will be "bag and masked". This involves placing a little plastic mask attached to a bag over her nose and mouth. The bag is squeezed to push air into the mask. This will hopefully get

> "I couldn't believe what was happening –
> it felt as though it was happening to someone else."
>
> *Dana, mum to Erin and Max*

will be covered up and dried so she stays warm and loses as little water through her skin as possible.

If it is a vaginal delivery, the resuscitaire is likely to be in the same room in which your baby is born. If you have a Caesarean section, it may be in the operating theatre or it could be in a little room next door. Wherever it is, it's always nearby. You will get to see your baby as soon as possible. If a mum is unable to watch what is going on, the dad will be able to tell her what's happening.

The moment the baby is born, a timer is started so that the medical team can record the baby's condition at precise times. The baby's heart rate, colour, oxygen requirements, and breathing are assessed at one minute, five minutes, and 10 minutes after the birth. This is known as the Apgar test. Each assessment is given a score between 0

the baby to take some breaths without having an endotracheal tube (see below) put in, and sometimes that's all a baby needs to get breathing started. She will then just breathe by herself.

Very premature babies who aren't able to breathe will need an endotracheal tube. This is a flexible tube that is inserted through the baby's mouth or nose, passed down through the trachea (windpipe) and between the vocal cords into the lungs, a process known as intubation. It means that oxygen or air can be administered directly into the lungs, which is called ventilation.

Without ventilation, a baby unable to breathe would die. The risk of a ventilator is that every breath you put in causes trauma to the baby's lungs, called "pressure trauma". The pressure applied can be reduced by administering surfactant, a substance that coats the air sacs in the lungs and prevents them from collapsing while breathing. Premature babies have little or no surfactant. Without it, the lungs will collapse again after air is introduced into them, and the inner surfaces of the lungs will stick together. This means that the pressure needed to open the lungs with the next breath is huge. One of the biggest revolutions in the care of premature babies has been the development of artificial surfactant. This is an opalescent, whitish liquid that comes in little vials.

After an endotracheal tube has been inserted, a few millilitres of surfactant are squirted into the lungs. This then dissipates as the baby is given breaths and the pressure in the lungs is reduced. As the lungs start to expand and work properly, it becomes much easier to ventilate the baby, the baby's oxygen requirement goes right down – and the medical team can start to relax.

Surfactant is given immediately in the delivery room if possible, and certainly all very premature babies are likely to be given it at this stage. Often, the nurses will have got the surfactant ready before the birth. As it's kept in the fridge, it needs to be warmed up to the right temperature.

It's very important to keep the baby warm throughout this process, so the resuscitaire has an overhead heater and the baby is kept wrapped up the whole time.

Into the neonatal unit
Once a baby is stable, the resuscitaire is wheeled into the neonatal unit and the baby is placed on the scales and weighed, which must be done very accurately. Dad can go with the baby, watch her being weighed, and take a quick photo to show to mum and the rest of the family.

After being weighed, the baby is placed into an incubator to keep her warm, and the monitoring and treatment process begins.

DAD'S EXPERIENCE
First moments

"The doctor said, 'Are you the daddy?' Then he said, 'Say hello to your son.'

They had this big heater machine, and he stood back, pressed the breathing pump, and all I saw was my son, face up in a clear see-through plastic bag, and you saw his chest expanding and going up every time they pressed the little button. I'll never forget the doctor. He had his back to me, and he had a shirt on, and all I saw was a sweat patch on his back, and I'll never forget that. In that one millisecond, I thought, 'Someone is going out of their way to save my baby'.**"**

Bal, dad to Leo

Resuscitaire A resuscitaire will be positioned near the mother during delivery. Once the baby is born, she will be placed on the resuscitaire to be checked over.

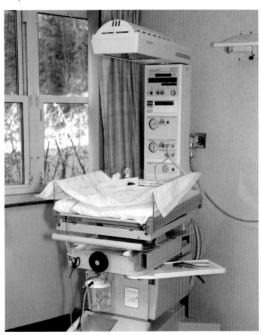

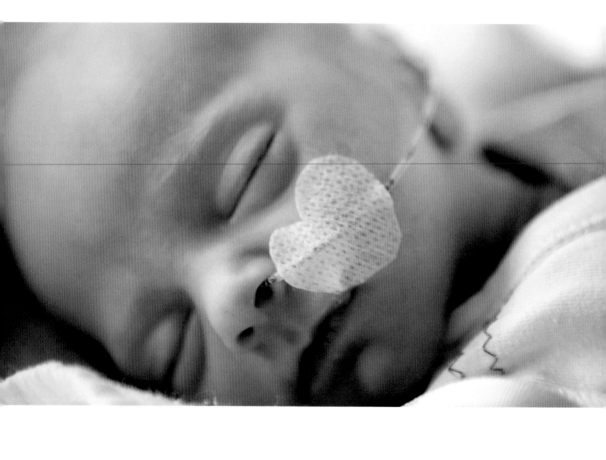

The neonatal unit

Going into the neonatal unit for the first time can be disturbing, but remember that everyone is intensely focused on doing the very best for your baby.

Arriving in the unit

Once your baby has been stabilized and settled into the neonatal unit, you'll be able to spend as much time there with her as you like. If she's well enough and you feel ready, you'll quickly be able to get involved in her care.

Parents should be able to go into the neonatal unit as soon as possible to be with their child. Dads can go in straight away with the medical team as the baby is wheeled through from the delivery room. That means he's there to watch his baby being weighed and can see her being put into the incubator. He can also take photos; there's no need to worry too much about the flash going off – the baby will blink a little bit but it won't hurt her. A lot of babies have their eyes closed at this point anyway. If dad takes pictures of his baby on his mobile phone, it means that he can send them to family and friends, and, more importantly, it means that if mum can't get to the unit straight away, she will have photos of her baby to look at.

Lots of units, especially more modern ones, have the labour ward next to the neonatal unit, which means that if there is space, a new mum can be wheeled into the unit on her bed. So even if you've just had a Caesarean, you may be able to see your baby on the neonatal unit very soon afterwards.

Doctors sometimes ask parents to step outside as there is often a frenzy of activity initially while a baby is being stabilized, and so they can concentrate on tricky procedures. One of the team can pop out and update both parents on how the baby is doing.

In the unit Even when your baby is in an incubator, you can hold her gently, but firmly, when she's stable enough. This will help her feel secure.

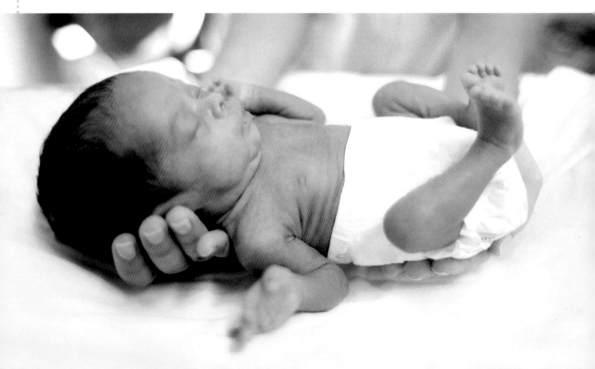

Transferring to other units If your local unit is unable to accommodate your baby, either because of lack of space or because your baby will need a greater level of intensive care than can be provided, she will need to be transferred to another unit where specialist care will be available.

Ideally, doctors always try to transfer the mum before the baby has been born. This is called an "in-utero" transfer. It allows for mother and baby to be together and is the safest method of transport for the baby. However, if your obstetrician thinks it would be unsafe for you to travel, your baby will be born locally. This is also the case if you suddenly have complications during pregnancy and your baby needs to be born immediately. Your baby will be looked after by the paediatricians until she can be collected by a special neonatal transport team and taken to the nearest available neonatal unit. Unfortunately, this can sometimes be a long way away. When she is stable, your baby will travel to the new unit in a special transport incubator, which can be plugged into all the facilities in the ambulance. Her oxygen levels and temperature can then be monitored for the entire journey.

Parents are not usually allowed to travel in the ambulance with their baby owing to lack of space, but they can travel separately and meet the baby at the neonatal unit. If a mum is too sick to be discharged from hospital, it may be possible for her care to be transferred to the new hospital if it is considered safe for her to travel. As soon as your baby is ready to return to your local neonatal unit this will be arranged.

Transitional care Some hospitals have a small ward as part of the neonatal unit or a special part of the postnatal ward for "transitional" care. These areas are where mums and babies can be looked after together if the baby needs extra nursing but not intensive care.

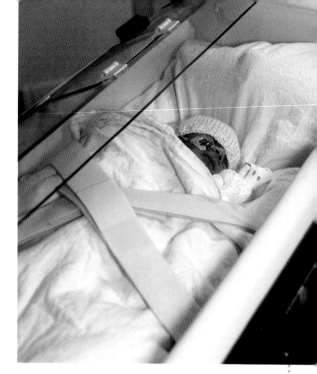

Special transfer If your baby has to be moved to another hospital, she'll be taken in a special transport incubator that enables her to be monitored and cared for while she travels.

DADS' EXPERIENCE
Without mum

"My wife was recovering from the Caesarean, and the normal thing is to take fathers in by themselves to meet their baby. There was a team of doctors so it was hard to get a private moment. Maybe if you were given a designated nurse to stand next to you and give you a hug – that would help."

Ross, dad to Freddie

"All I wanted to know at first was would he be okay. The consultants and nurses would talk medically about his condition, but nothing was sinking in. I just wanted to know if everything was going to be okay."

Nick, dad to Xavier

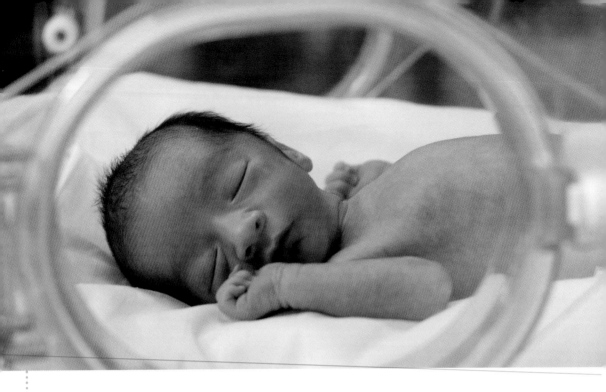

First impressions

If you've never been on a neonatal unit, the unfamiliar sights and sounds can be overwhelming at first. However, rest assured that all the equipment is there to help the medical team give your baby the best possible start in life.

Despite enormous advances in neonatal care, nothing can replace the womb in terms of support for a growing, developing fetus. Every effort is made in the unit to provide the best possible environment and care for each baby, but it can be quite daunting to see rows of incubators and scary-looking machines.

If you've never been into a neonatal unit before, you'll discover a whole new world with its own language, sounds, and rhythm. All the staff and everything that happens in the unit are intensely focused on doing the very best for each and every baby who arrives there.

If you know your baby is likely to need admission to the unit when he's born, it really is worthwhile to have a look round before the birth. A visit will give you an idea about what to expect when your baby arrives and allay some of your fears. A nurse will be able to show you around the unit and explain everything you'll need to know, and answer any questions you may have.

Hopefully you'll notice a quiet atmosphere, as it's known that babies thrive in a calm environment. Everything is deliberately toned down to mimic the womb as much as possible. While this can never be as effective as the womb, you may see padded covers

New world Your baby's incubator will be kept quiet and dimly lit so he can rest and grow. The portholes allow access for care while disturbing him as little as possible.

over the incubators, which help to insulate the baby from light and sound (see p.29), and the staff will try to talk softly and carry out tasks quietly to disturb the babies as little as possible.

Generally all you'll hear is the beeping of the monitors or occasional flurries of activity when

baby when another baby comes in or becomes unwell, you may be asked to wait outside, just as when your baby needs attention, other parents may be asked to leave. Confidentiality is very important in healthcare and this starts from the very beginning of life. Even the tiniest of patients needs respect, as do his parents. If you are asked to leave, take advantage of the time to have a break and a cup of tea and chat to other parents.

> " It's a whole world in here. It prepares and protects you, and gives you the foundations to face the real world. "
>
> *Bal, dad to Leo*

there's an emergency. Everyone is as careful as they can be to keep things calm and quiet. If someone does make a sudden noise, you may see the babies all startle.

Sometimes the unit can get very busy when a new baby is being admitted or if a baby suddenly needs attention. If you are on the unit with your

There's a lot to take in when you first see the unit and all the equipment, and it can be an overwhelming experience, so don't hesitate to ask questions – even if they're the same questions over and over again – as often as you need to. The medical staff know this is a trying time and will answer all your questions if they can.

MY STORY

Dana says...

" After Erin was born they took her to the neonatal ward when she was stable. Once I'd come to a little, they wheeled me in to see her. I hadn't even come round really – I couldn't walk and I was in a bit of a state.

I was just so scared of everything that was going on in the neonatal unit: the beeps, the machines, the alarms, and the flashing lights.

She was in the incubator with wires and tubes coming out every which way, and there was also the ventilator, and it was just heartbreaking. I thought,

'Is that my baby?' You just couldn't believe a baby could be so small.

Then the next day, I went in there for the first time after having some sleep, and she had the de-sats, where the oxygen saturation levels go down, and also bradycardia, where the heartbeat is too slow. Her breathing stopped, basically. The staff literally had to remind her to breathe. When that happened, I just left the room. I couldn't cope with the situation. I felt so guilty that I was running away and not staying and helping my baby, but there was nothing I could do. My baby had stopped breathing and that's all I saw. "

Dana, mum to Erin and Max

How is the unit organized?

Where your baby will stay in the unit will depend on how much care she needs. Every unit is slightly different, but all will be as quiet and dimly lit as possible to ensure a peaceful environment for your baby.

Neonatal units vary across the country and around the world, but however they are structured, their role is to provide the best-quality care for premature and sick babies.

Some units will have 50 intensive care cots, while others may have as few as six. Some units do not have intensive care at all, but will send the smallest

Levels of care Once your baby is born, she may be taken to one of three different types of neonatal unit, which each offer different levels of care.

Level one Sometimes also called the special care baby unit (SCBU), level one is for babies who require extra care, such as oxygen or nasogastric feeds, but who don't need ventilation.

> "In intensive care you're so freaked out you might not speak to anyone except the nurses, but by the time you're ready to go home, you've almost got used to it."
>
> *Carolyn, mum to Evie*

and sickest babies to a more specialist centre, and the babies will then return when they are bigger and more stable. If your baby is born at a hospital that specializes in intensive care, but she doesn't need that level of intervention, she may be moved to a different hospital to free up an intensive care bed for a sicker baby.

The health professionals who carry out procedures will also vary. In many intensive care units, advanced nurse practitioners will be responsible for carrying out roles that in other units would be performed by junior doctors. Rest assured that whoever is looking after your baby will have all the necessary training and experience to give her the very best quality of care. It's good to know, too, that if you are not at the hospital, you can phone the neonatal unit at any time, day or night, to ask the staff how your baby is doing.

Level two These units are able to care for babies who need extra help with their breathing or specialist intravenous feeds, but who are expected to recover quickly.

Level three Babies who are taken to level three require very specialist intensive care; these include premature babies born at less than 27 weeks or babies who need neonatal surgery.

Special rooms Within a level two or three unit there will be different sections to cater for babies with greater or lesser needs. These sections, or rooms, are sometimes called "hot", "warm", and "cool" rooms to denote how much care the babies in them need, not the temperature of the room. The hot room, also called intensive care, is the section for the sickest babies, who need ventilators and extra attention. As a baby gets better and stronger, she will be moved out of intensive care into the

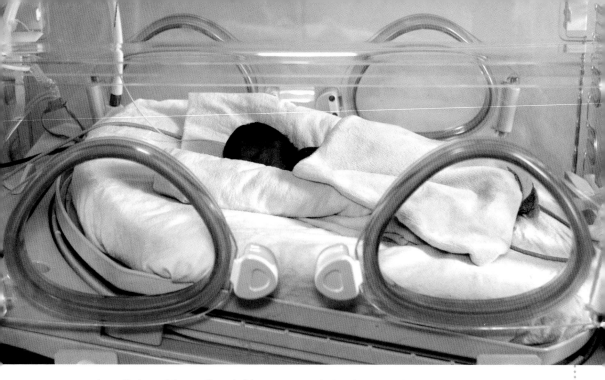

warm room, also called special care. Once babies are in the cool room, they will be getting used to feeding and gaining weight, ready to go home. It's in here that you'll be learning everything you'll need to know about caring for your baby before you take her home.

Light and sound
Recently, a lot of research has focused on how the environment in the neonatal unit can be improved. It has shown that if babies are nursed in low light with minimal noise they are likely to go home sooner and to grow faster and need less oxygen. You may notice in your baby's unit that the nurses keep the lights dimmed and may put covers over the incubators to block out any harsh lighting.

Constant bright lights aren't good for your baby's eyes, even when they are closed. When she's very premature and if the lights are on all the time, this can disrupt her natural body rhythms.

The medical team may turn the lights on when it's time for ward rounds or they need to examine your baby at another time. They will protect your

In the incubator Your baby may look very tiny inside her incubator but this is the best place for her to receive the care she needs and continue to develop and grow.

baby's eyes, where possible, when they need to use a bright light for examinations.

If your baby is in a closed incubator with a cover, keep the cover on and lift the flap to talk softly or sing to her. Use the individual light next to the cot or incubator and avoid shining it in your baby's eyes.

Premature babies can be very sensitive to sound so it's important to remember to carry out simple tasks quietly. For example, if you put things on top of your baby's incubator, put them down gently to avoid making a noise, which is amplified in a closed space, and remember to close the lids of rubbish bins quietly if you use them. The nursing staff can decrease the alarm levels on the monitors where possible, and everyone makes an effort to avoid making loud, sudden noises as much as they can. There may be notices around the unit, reminding everyone to be quiet.

Equipment you may see on the unit

It can be frightening to see your baby attached to various bits of kit by different lines and tubes. However, this equipment is vital to monitor his progress and give him any support or treatment he needs.

Equipment that you may see in the neonatal unit is likely to include some or all of the following.

Incubator On your baby's arrival, he will be placed in an incubator, which is a special cot where he can be kept warm and that allows staff easy access to administer treatment. In some units, very unstable babies may be placed in an open incubator with an overhead heater, so there is easy access all the time. Most babies, though, are nursed in a closed incubator, which is covered and has portholes for access. Premature babies lose a lot of water through their skin and an open incubator isn't good

for maintaining humidity. If a baby has been placed in an open incubator, he'll be moved to a closed incubator once he is stable enough

Ventilator If a baby needs help to breathe, an endotracheal tube is inserted (see p.20) through the nose or mouth, and attached to a ventilator, which blows air or oxygen into the lungs. The amount of oxygen can be modified according to the baby's needs. In an emergency, the tube will be inserted immediately with no sedation, but if there is time, the baby can be given drugs to sedate and relax him to prepare him for insertion of the tube.

Ventilator If your baby needs a lot of support with breathing, a ventilator can breathe for him. A tube in his trachea (windpipe) delivers oxygen directly into his lungs.

CPAP A baby who needs extra help with breathing may be given CPAP. This works by puffing air into his nose to support his breathing without needing to use a ventilator.

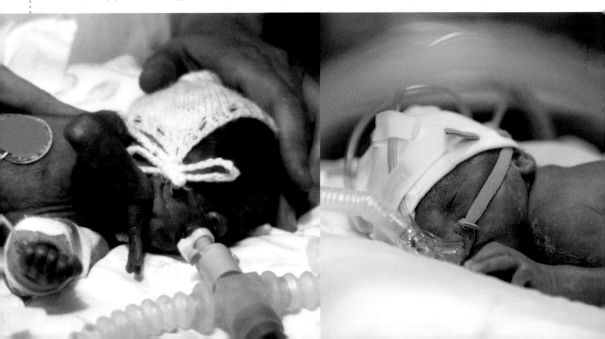

Continuous positive airways pressure (CPAP)

If a baby can breathe but is tiring easily or having episodes when breathing stops (apnoea), CPAP can support breathing without the need to intubate. It is applied via prongs that fit into the baby's nose. They have to fit well with a tight seal so that the CPAP machine can deliver air or oxygen under pressure to the lungs. The pressure helps prevent the lungs collapsing between breaths.

Infusion pumps

All babies in intensive care will have fluids and drugs delivered at the correct rate by a number of pumps.

Cannula

This fine tube goes into a vein. It is used to take blood for testing or to deliver fluids and/or drugs, procedures needed by virtually every baby coming into a neonatal unit. The cannula comes with a fine needle inside it. The needle is removed once the cannula has been placed in the vein.

Cannula This tiny tube is inserted into a baby's vein for taking blood or giving fluids and/or medicine. Here, the doctor has inserted a cannula and is taking a blood sample.

Long line

This very fine, flexible tube is threaded along a vein almost into the heart and used to give liquid nourishment to babies who cannot digest as much milk as they need. For most small babies milk will not be enough, and they will receive fluid called total parenteral nutrition (TPN) for the first few days or weeks (see p.62).

Suction

When a baby has a lot of secretions in his mouth or nose, the nurse will use a suction pump to remove them.

Saturation monitor

This is a handy way of constantly assessing the amount of oxygen in the baby's blood. A probe wrapped around the baby's foot or hand detects oxygen levels through the skin.

Cerebral function monitor (CFM)

This monitor may be put on to a baby's head to assess whether or not the baby is having fits (seizures).

Saturation monitor This sensor is attached to the baby's hand or foot and shines a light through his skin to show how much oxygen is being carried by the blood.

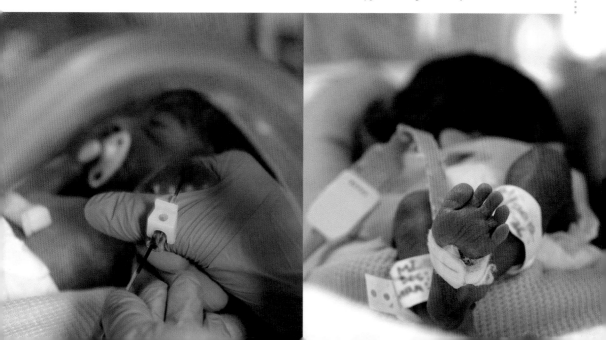

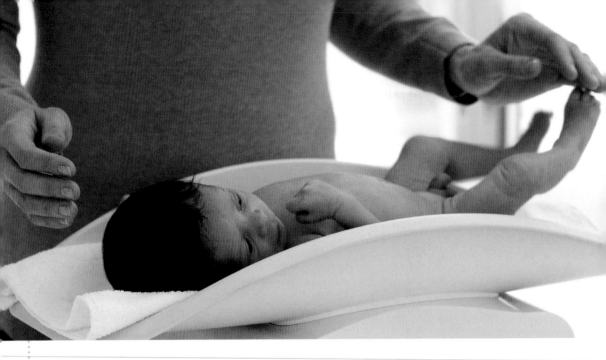

Daily routines

The medical team will monitor your baby carefully during her stay in the neonatal unit. The doctors and nurses caring for her will give you regular updates on her progress and will tell you if she needs any further treatment.

Every unit has a daily ward round during which the medical team sees each baby in turn. Before the ward round, the night staff will update the day team about each baby in a detailed handover.

Generally, there will be regular updates from the nursing staff and junior doctors along with intermittent meetings with the consultant paediatrician. A consultant paediatrician who specializes in providing intensive care to newborn babies is known as a neonatologist. If you have an immediate worry, talk to the nurse looking after your baby. There is also always a doctor available in the unit. There will be several consultants in charge of the neonatal unit and in most units there will be one consultant, called the "attending consultant",

each week with responsibility for the day-to-day care of all the babies. So although your baby may have a named consultant, her day-to-day care will be shared between consultants. Exactly how this works will depend on the individual hospital.

All units have 24-hour access for families and if you're not in the hospital you can call at any time, night or day. It's important that you feel able to speak with the consultant when you're worried or want to discuss your baby's progress.

Ward rounds Most neonatal units have one main ward round per day and often smaller ward rounds at handover times. The team, usually led by the consultant, will discuss all the details about each

Reaching a healthy weight Your baby will be weighed regularly while he's on the unit to check he is gaining weight and growing as expected.

baby and will examine each baby, and then make a plan for the next few hours or day.

You may be invited to be there while your baby is discussed, but you'll be asked to leave while they discuss the other babies. If the unit doesn't allow parents to be present during the ward round, the medical team will update you about your baby's progress and answer any questions you may have.

The discussions about each baby are usually very detailed and technical and can sound like a different language. For some parents, being involved in these discussions can feel helpful; for others, it is overwhelming and frightening. Even if your baby's unit allows parents to be present during ward rounds, you may still prefer to wait until the end of the round and ask the nurse or doctor to update you – or you may feel reassured by being present throughout and being able to ask questions as your baby's treatment is being discussed.

However things work in your unit, it's very important that you feel able to ask questions and that you are updated regularly. It will be hard to leave your baby and go home (see p.42), but the staff will always phone you if they are worried about your baby, any time of day or night. They will also update you whenever you phone, so if you're lying in bed at night and worrying about your baby, just phone to be reassured.

Your baby's medical records
The doctors and nurses will keep detailed notes about your baby's progress. Units may have slightly different ways of doing this, but in general the nurses will write any observations on a large chart that is next to the incubator and is updated at least every four hours. The doctors write their notes in a folder,

which is usually kept in a trolley. Entries are made in these notes during ward rounds and whenever there are any significant changes noted in your baby or a procedure is carried out.

Hygiene
Babies on the unit are very vulnerable to infection, partly because their immune systems are immature and can't fight off infections well. In addition, life-saving intensive care techniques they may need, such as intubation or insertion of a long line for total parenteral nutrition (TPN) (see p.62), increase the risk of infection.

Before entering the unit, you and any visitors must wash their hands and use the alcohol gel provided. Watches and any large rings and bracelets must be removed, and sleeves rolled up. If you or a visitor has a tummy upset, cold, or any other bug, speak to the staff first so they can advise on the best thing to do.

You'll usually be asked not to bring children into the unit apart from your baby's brothers and sisters to keep the risk of infection to a minimum, and most units ask that there are not more than two visitors at a time by each incubator or cot, one of which should be a parent.

TIPS

Parents say...

"Live day to day. People would ask how Leo was and say you must be looking forward to taking him home. We'd reply we just live day to day."

Bal, dad to Leo

"Talk to other parents on the unit. I found it really useful. It was good to share stories and to know that we were not alone with our experience."

Kamini, mum to Jaden

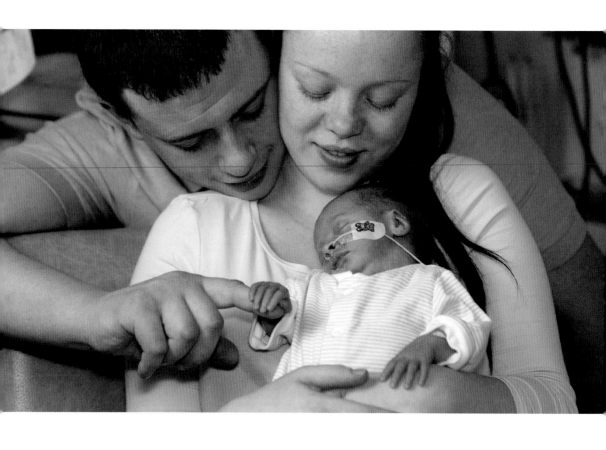

Life on the unit

You'll soon adjust to the high-tech atmosphere of the neonatal unit and find a way to start building a relationship with your baby.

How you may feel

It's normal to go through emotional ups and downs while your baby is on the neonatal unit, and it's important to lean on family and friends. If you're struggling with your feelings, talk to the staff, who can offer you extra support.

When your baby arrives on the neonatal unit, you may feel that your whole world has been turned upside-down. This is not what you expected the early days with your new baby to be like, and you may feel anxious, exhausted, bewildered, overwhelmed, without a role, distanced from your baby, depressed, scared, and full of questions. You may feel proud to be parents but not sure whether to tell anyone or what to say to friends who phone.

The unit may seem alien, clinical, mechanical, and technical, with lots of unfamiliar noises from monitors and alarms, and if your baby is very premature you may be terrified that even all that technology still won't be able to keep your tiny baby alive. It's normal to feel shocked at the size of your baby if he's arrived early.

You might worry that your baby may get cold if he's in an open incubator and be scared that you won't know how to communicate with him. Parents are often distressed that they might be unable to touch or hold their baby without upsetting him, and it is usual to feel self-conscious, unsure, and insecure.

Mums and dads Parents may each feel very different. Mums often focus on the baby – how he looks, whether he's calm or irritable – and tend to ask about feeds and cuddles. Dads frequently want to learn how to assess how their baby is doing by looking at numbers on monitors; they often ask about technical details and blood results and become very interested in the technology. Both outlooks are important and the staff will try to guide and support you in coming to terms with what is happening and what role you can play.

Mum and dad can both get involved with the practical care of their baby – washing and nappy-changing, for instance. If a dad has to go back to work early on, a mum may be on the unit more during the day; if a dad is going to be the main carer for the baby, he may spend more time doing the practical care. Every family is different.

Getting support This is a very difficult time and can be an emotional roller coaster for parents. The intense worry and stress of having a baby on the neonatal unit can put a huge strain on the

> "I've got into a bad habit. Whenever I come in I just look at the machine. That's how I know my son."
> *Bal, dad to Leo*

strongest of relationships, and sometimes, sadly, couples even split up as a result.

Most neonatal units will offer emotional support for parents. This may include counsellors, specialist nurses, psychiatrists, and psychotherapists. You can also speak to your doctor or midwife. Depending on the hospital your baby is in, there may be the opportunity to get together with other parents so you can share your experiences. Various charities offer support, counselling, advice, and even arrange parent groups (see p.124 for useful resources).

Postnatal depression

This condition affects around one in every 10 mums, and it is considerably more common when your baby has been born prematurely. It often starts within a month of your baby's birth, but it can happen any time in the first year. Postnatal depression is not the same as "baby blues", which usually starts around the fourth day after giving birth and lasts for a few days. If you have any of the following symptoms most of the time for a period of two weeks, you could be suffering from postnatal depression:

- Feeling low
- Irritability
- Anxiety
- Tearfulness
- Difficulty concentrating
- Feelings of negativity
- Not being able to bond with your baby
- Inability to cope
- Loss of appetite
- Difficulty sleeping
- Panic attacks.

While it's natural to feel overwhelmed when you have a baby who needs special care, if you're struggling with how you are feeling it's important to seek help and support as soon as you can. In milder cases, postnatal depression can pass in a few months with some emotional and practical support. However, in more severe cases, extra help in the form of counselling and/or medication may be necessary, and you might be referred to a crisis team. Postnatal depression responds very well to these treatments and you should never hesitate to seek help. If not treated, the problem can persist and can have a serious effect on your life, as well as on your family and those around you.

see p.124 for useful resources

MY STORY

Carolyn says...

"When Evie was born, I was completely numb. I was just trying to keep it together. I felt like I was never going to walk again, I was never going to be well, and it had all gone so horribly wrong. But I was desperately trying not to panic.

For two weeks I was okay and then it started. I felt I couldn't cope and that I couldn't leave the hospital. I just wanted someone to look after me.

I couldn't sleep or eat and, of course, you can't make milk without eating. I just thought, 'I am useless and pathetic and I can't deal with this.'

I found I couldn't leave the parents' room. I just wanted to stay in there. I was panicking, panicking, panicking. The staff had obviously spotted it as Matron came in and said, 'What can we do for you?' I told them I needed help and they got me an emergency referral.

They said I had probably been depressed during pregnancy and that I was now also suffering from postnatal depression and post-traumatic stress – everything, really. There were counsellors who I could meet every day, and also a phone number I could ring whenever I needed. It was a lifeline.

I just wanted someone to say, 'You'll get better', and I needed to hear it every day, every hour. I was able to call someone and say, 'I'm not going to get better, I thought I was getting better but now I feel worse,' and someone would say, 'You will get better, we've seen this before.' They also got involved in my long-term care and came to see me at home. I was put on medication and, gradually, it just got better.

I feel embarrassed having to take antidepressants in order to function, although I know I shouldn't be as lots of people take them. I'm very lucky that they help me. Now I'm like I used to be.**"**

Carolyn, mum to Evie

Working with the medical team

Although your baby's care will be led by a highly experienced medical and nursing team, they will want you to work in partnership with them and to understand what is happening throughout your baby's stay on the unit.

The care of your baby is a partnership between you and the staff. Important decisions will be discussed with you, and the nurses and doctors are there to support you through all the ups and downs. No treatment is without risk and treatments are always offered because it is felt that the benefit significantly outweighs the risk. For example, ventilating a baby puts her at risk of chronic lung disease, but not ventilating a baby who cannot breathe by herself means that she would die.

responsibility for how it is run. The most junior doctors on the unit, known as senior house officers (SHOs), will have trained for a minimum of eight years. They are supervised by registrars, who are a lot more experienced.

The more you understand about your baby's treatment the better, but sometimes parents feel they have learned so much that they start suggesting technical changes, such as to ventilation or oxygen levels. While it's important for you to feel

> "The nurses would never let the conversation get beyond what was happening at that moment. They'd say, 'You can't worry about tomorrow.'"
>
> *Bal, dad to Leo*

It's important that you fully understand your baby's treatment. Ask for an interpreter if you need one. Everyone must work together to ensure that your baby receives the best medical support as well as all the love and nurturing that she needs.

When you first arrive on the unit, you'll meet lots of doctors and nurses and it can be very difficult to remember everyone. The nurses are all expertly trained and will provide your baby with day-to-day care. Nurses will also show you how to look after her. The matron has overall responsibility for the nurses and manages the unit. Sisters and charge nurses are the most senior after the matron, followed by staff nurses. The consultant paediatrician is the most senior doctor working on the unit and, along with the matron, has overall

confident that the medical team is taking good care of your baby, suggesting alternatives to your baby's care is beyond your role, which is to be her parents, not her nurses or doctors.

Some parents develop a particularly close working relationship with certain nurses, but it is not practical to demand that your baby be looked after by particular nurses. However, it is important that you feel comfortable and happy with your baby's care, so if you have a serious concern, do ask to speak to a senior nurse or doctor. Once you raise them, misunderstandings can easily be cleared up.

Caring together Your baby's consultant will be happy to spend time updating you on her progress and will answer any questions you may have.

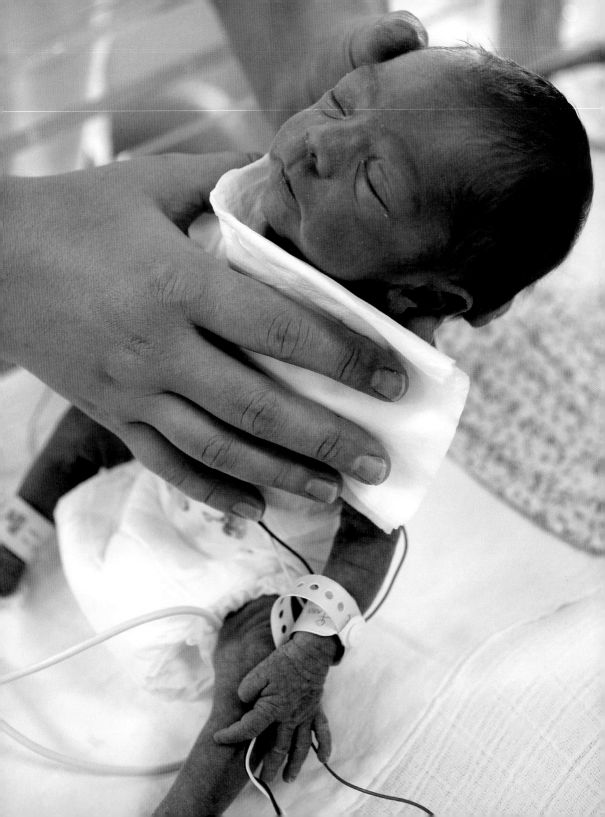

Your role on the unit

Parents are very important people on the unit and there are lots of things you'll be able to do for your baby, depending on how stable he is. Don't worry – you will be shown what to do and you'll have all the help you need.

You have a vital role as your baby's mum or dad. Some parents find it very hard to get too involved at first as the situation can feel so uncertain. Also, many parents feel helpless in the face of so much used to parents who find it difficult to even step into the unit at first, but they will have lots of ideas for ways to help you. As the minutes, hours, and days go by and your baby seems stronger, you may

> **"**We held his hands, we stroked his head, we sang to him, we spoke to him, we prayed.**"**
>
> *Dana, mum to Erin and Max*

medical technology, but remember that you are the most important people to your baby.

Mums and dads can also be scared to bond with their baby in case he dies. The medical team will understand this and will encourage you to spend time with him from the very beginning. They are become more confident and allow yourself to start bonding with him. One day, when you look at this

Loving touch These twins take comfort from being together. Touch, sounds, and smell are all important to your baby and he'll be reassured by a familiar presence.

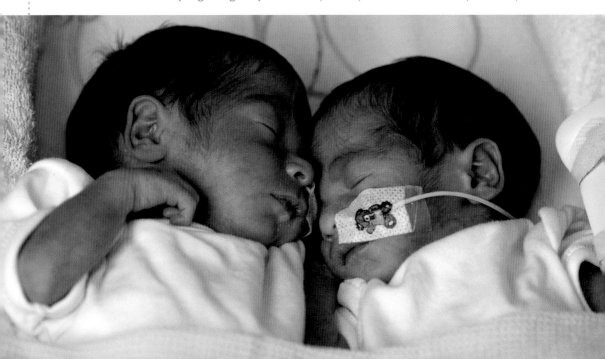

tiny, vulnerable being in his incubator, you'll find yourself falling in love and realizing that whatever happens in the future, you will always be his parent.

You may discover that you have a strong preference for what you would like to be called by the nurses and doctors. Whether this is "mum", "dad" or your first name, it's fine to let them know.

Why you're important As your baby's parents, you can offer him continuity of care and you can help him feel less stressed in the hospital environment. However well the nurses wash him or change his nappy, they work different shifts, have days off, and go on holiday, but you're always there for your baby – and you're never the ones to cause discomfort if he needs blood taken or a tube put in.

Very early on, babies begin to relax when their parents arrive on the unit. Their heart rates actually settle when they hear mum's or dad's voice or feel their touch. Even if you have a very tiny, very premature baby, he will get to know you quickly, which is lovely for him and lovely for you. He is beginning to understand that he isn't alone and that you are a source of comfort.

As your baby grows bigger, you'll be able to do more for him. The nurses will show you how to take on aspects of your baby's practical care, such as changing his nappy, cleaning his face, and eventually bathing him (see pp.54–57). You'll also be able to hold the syringe for tube feeds, breastfeed him when he's able to suck, and cuddle him when he's stable enough (see Kangaroo care, p.58).

You're a very important part of a team – the team caring for your baby. When there are key decisions to be made about your baby's care, you'll be fully informed and consulted and the medical team will ensure that they explain everything to you. Your role in this is to ask if you haven't understood anything, as staff will always be happy to explain what's happening as many times as needed.

MY STORY
Sophie says...

"There was a part of me that held back in the beginning. I was so scared I was going to lose them that I didn't want to give myself entirely to them. But now they've got me 100 per cent. It's been really hard. They were born at 26 weeks, but Samuel's gone up and up, whereas Leo has struggled. Ever since Leo was born, he's had infections, one after the other, so it was a bit touch and go with him in the beginning. He was nil by mouth for a long time, which meant his brother had a head start on weight – on everything really.

Leo was on ventilation for a while, whereas Samuel wasn't. Samuel was ventilated for one day, then moved onto a nasal cannula with a bit of air flow as well as oxygen – not just oxygen. And then about three weeks ago they said, 'Let's see how he does on his own', and that was that. He's never really needed any breathing help at all.

With Leo, it's the complete opposite. He really needs it, and he's got really weak lungs.

They said Leo will take a long time to become stronger and that's what made my decision to take Samuel home. The plan is to bring Samuel with me when I come to see Leo. I'm more nervous about this than if both of them were coming home. But Samuel's well and I've got an overriding feeling that he should be home when he's strong enough. He's not going to thrive here; he needs to be at home. It's not an easy option for me: the easy option would be to keep them together and take them home when they're both ready. A lot of mums with twins do keep them in hospital together, but I think that development-wise, they're so far apart, it's just not fair on Samuel if he stays in for longer. **"**

Sophie, mum to Samuel and Leo

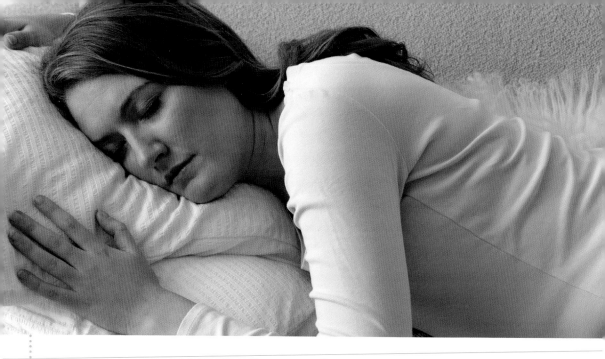

Leaving your baby in hospital

Your baby may need to spend weeks or even months in the neonatal unit and leaving her there when you go home will be very hard. It can be difficult to get on with everyday life, but you can ring for an update at any time.

It can be very hard when it's time for you to go home, but your baby isn't ready to leave hospital with you. Tearing yourself away from your baby and not being there all the time can feel devastating. Returning to an empty house with everything set up to receive your new baby seems totally wrong. If you have another child, it may feel important to get home as quickly as possible. This is particularly difficult if the unit is a long way from your home and you know that you won't be able to return quickly if necessary.

As a mum, you will be discharged as soon as the midwives say you are fit to go home. If your baby is very sick you may be able to stay a little longer if there's space for you, either on the postnatal ward or in a parents' room in the neonatal unit. However, space is often very limited, and if your baby is likely to spend several weeks in the unit, it will be much better for your strength and your sanity for you to be based at home and visit your baby in the unit every day for as long as possible.

Taking care of yourself You'll need to get as much rest and sleep as possible, eat well, and, if possible, express your breast milk every three to four hours regularly around the clock. Expressing milk is very important for your baby, even though it may be difficult to get the milk to flow initially if your baby was very premature. You are likely to get more sleep at home than in the unit, despite all the

Regaining your strength Although it will be incredibly hard to leave your baby on the unit, it is important you take care of yourself, so you can remain strong for her.

worry, but it's important to remember to set your alarm at night so that you can wake up to express milk. You can always phone the unit for an update while you're expressing!

Managing day by day You may have days when you struggle to deal with what's happening and this is completely normal. Ups and downs can happen at different stages for each parent and it's important for you to support each other as much

through. Eventually, you will find yourself offering the same kind of support to other parents. Many mums and dads make life-long friendships while their babies are on the unit.

Your friends and family will often ask what they can do to help. Don't hesitate to ask for what you need. This may include a listening ear, a shoulder to cry on, a lift to the hospital, baby-sitting for older children, or some home-cooked food. Sometimes you may just need a hug.

Parents often say that having a baby on the neonatal unit is an intensely emotional and very draining experience. You may find you're exhausted much of the time. Therefore it's very important to

> " I felt very guilty leaving him on his own. Obviously he was in safe hands, but I just wanted to be with him. "
>
> *Claudia, mum to Chase*

as you can. This is an incredibly stressful time for all mums and dads and, sadly, some relationships don't survive. For single parents, the support of friends and family will similarly be essential, both practically and emotionally.

Don't be afraid to speak to the other parents on the unit, who are going through a similar experience themselves. In the early days, it can be a huge relief to talk to people who know the ropes, and they'll often be only too happy to share their experiences with you. This can be in an informal way, such as meeting for a coffee after you've been to see your babies, or in a more formal setting with a group of other parents, such as a neonatal drop-in session arranged by the hospital.

No matter how many questions you ask the medical team and how well-informed you are, the doctors and nurses aren't experiencing this from a parents' perspective and you'll find it really helps to talk with people who understand what you're going

get away from the hospital sometimes. Try to spend time with your partner, family, and friends doing normal, everyday things, even though it feels as though part of your life is on hold. A meal out, seeing a film, and playing with your older children are all important too.

> TIPS
> ## Parents say...
>
> " Take people's support and get out whenever you can. You have to maintain a little bit of the outside world; otherwise, you lose touch. "
>
> *Claudia, mum to Chase*
>
> " Spend time with your partner away from the hospital. You still need time together. "
>
> *Cher, mum to Xavier*

Siblings and other people

If your baby has arrived early or is ill and has to stay in hospital, older children may feel jealous or worried, and your reassurance is vital. Telling others about the situation can be hard; it may help to send a group email or start a blog.

Siblings It's very difficult if you have other children because you may want to spend all day with your new baby. Check whether the hospital allows you to bring your older children onto the unit for a visit. It's not always easy to have them

Siblings' reactions may depend on how premature your baby is, or what level of treatment he currently needs. Seeing their new brother or sister attached to lots of tubes and wires and hearing the sounds from the machines can be puzzling for young children,

> " I really missed the whole fanfare of when you bring a baby home. People didn't know how to behave. You've had a baby, but no one celebrated anything. "
>
> *Carolyn, mum to Evie*

at the hospital for long periods of time, as they are likely to get bored and to need your attention. If you can, get a friend to bring them in and then take them home after a while.

Brothers and sisters However worried you are, it's important to spend time playing with your other children as they need to know that you're still there for them.

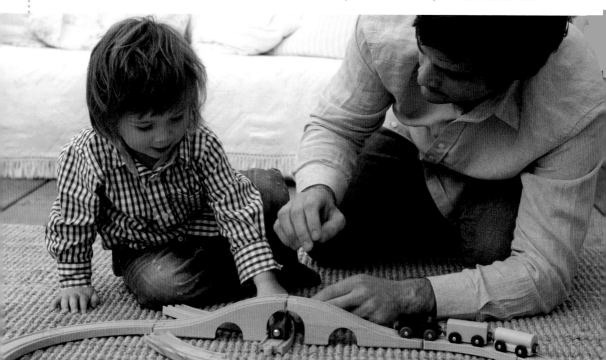

although many take it in their stride. Explain simply what a few of the tubes are for and how they are helping the baby. Siblings may only be able to look at the baby through the incubator, but if your baby is well enough, then his more grown-up siblings may be able to touch him.

It is quite common for an older brother or sister to feel jealous and resentful of how much attention their new sibling is receiving – especially if you are having to travel for a large amount of time each day. Try to keep their routine as consistent as possible, and keep reassuring them that although you have to spend a lot of your time with the new baby, you have just as much love and concern for them.

Older children may also understand a little of what is happening and feel the worry and stress felt by parents. If your children do understand aspects of the situation, then speak to them about it and answer honestly any questions they may have.

Depending on their ages, you can try to involve your other children in your baby's care. For example, they can read or talk to your baby if he is in an

will upset or offend you. A new baby is cause for celebration, but people may worry that they're being insensitive if they send a congratulations card, or may agonize over what is an appropriate gift, or whether a gift is appropriate at all. Friends and

> "We were so conscious Samuel was also living this nightmare. It's vital to keep siblings' routines the same as it shows them that they're just as important. "
>
> *Cher, mum to Xavier*

incubator. Helping care for their brother or sister will encourage bonding and will also make siblings feel important. It may encourage them to help out when you bring your baby home.

Other people's reactions When you announce the arrival of a premature or very sick baby, people often don't know how to react. Do they congratulate you or commiserate with you? They will be both happy and concerned for you and your baby, but they may not know if a certain reaction

family may not want to intrude, or may think you might not want to speak to them about the situation. You may want to discuss every single detail of your baby to anyone who will listen. Or you may find it difficult to open up about him and struggle with what and how much you should tell others. Although this is a very difficult and worrying time, try to update people when you can. It may be easier to send an email with any news. This keeps people updated and also lets them know that you are grateful for their concern.

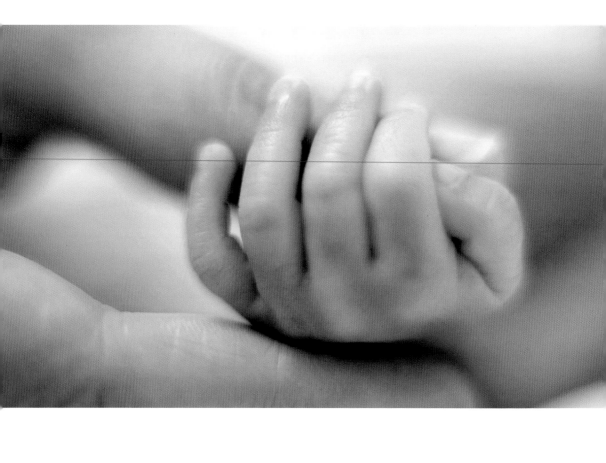

Caring for your baby

It is natural to feel nervous about handling your new baby at first, but she will quickly grow to recognize your touch and be comforted by your presence.

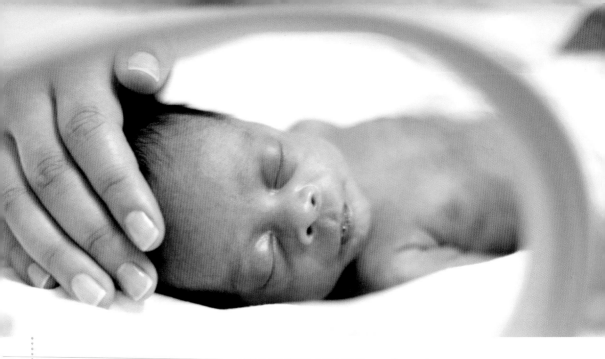

How do premature babies behave?

Your baby will be a tiny individual from the very start. You'll also notice that her behaviour depends on her stage of development, as well as on any medical issues that she may have.

You can't really know how your baby feels on leaving the cosy, warm environment of your womb and facing bright lights, noises, and all the procedures and treatments that have to be performed to keep her alive and healthy: you can only imagine.

Having a baby on the neonatal unit is not what you envisaged when you became pregnant. If your baby is born early and/or with medical problems, your expectations will have completely changed and you may feel there is nothing you can contribute to looking after her. However, even the sickest and most premature babies will benefit from their parents' care and attention.

When a baby is born at term, she can see, hear, feel, taste, and touch, and she will have a number of reflexes, including rooting (in which a baby will turn her head towards a touch on the cheek in search of the breast) and sucking. If a baby is born early, what she can do, how she will behave, her senses, and the reflexes she has will depend on how premature she is, and her individual development.

Sleep Premature babies usually sleep more than babies born at term. They can sleep for up to 20 hours a day. Doctors in the unit can examine babies from top to toe, then settle them down again and they go straight back to sleep! Because there are routines on the neonatal unit, babies often learn to sleep and feed in a regular pattern, which can make things easier when you get them home.

Slowly and gently Premature babies sleep for much of the time while they grow, mature, and adjust to the shock of life outside the womb.

Sight

If your baby is born early, her sight is still progressing and maturing, and is one of the last senses to develop. Although some visual stimulation is important, continuous bright light is not good for she is born, and talking or singing to her will be good for both of you. If she is in a closed incubator, open the portholes if you can so that your voice isn't distorted. When holding your baby close, the sound of your heartbeat, familiar to her from her time in the womb, will help to soothe and relax her. Sudden loud noises, such as monitor bleeps, alarms, telephones, and raised voices can be very

> **"I spent hours looking into his eyes. They say eyes are the windows to the soul and with Chase, that was very true."**
>
> *Claudia, mum to Chase*

her as her eyelids are thin and provide little protection. This is why the lights are kept low in neonatal units and often the incubators are covered. The eyelids of extremely premature babies may still be fused shut. They will gradually open in the first days or weeks. By 28 weeks, however, they'll be wide open and she will soon love focusing on your face.

Don't be alarmed if your baby's eyes don't look completely centred. Many term babies have the same problem, and their eyes don't coordinate fully until they are a few months old. Premature babies are at risk of a potentially serious eye problem known as retinopathy of prematurity (ROP) that can affect their sight, so she will be checked and monitored for this (see p.72).

Give your baby plenty of opportunities to look at your face. You can put photos on the inside of her cot so she will see your face when you're not there.

Sound

Nurses tend to chat to babies on the unit all the time, but parents are often amazed at first to know that their premature baby can hear. Her hearing developed in the womb, where she listened to your heartbeat, your blood flow, and also your voice. So she will already recognize your voice when stressful for your baby, and the medical team looking after her will try to avoid these as much as possible. If your baby is startled by a noise, the gentle sound of your familiar voice will help to calm and reassure her.

Tiny dummies Special dummies that are the right size for premature babies allow them to practise sucking for when they're able to feed from the breast or bottle.

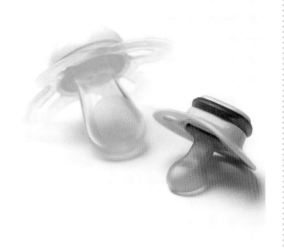

Sucking Although very premature babies have not yet developed a coordinated sucking reflex, your baby may like to have her hands close to her face, and once she is able to suck, she might put a finger in her mouth for comfort. Nurses on the unit may give her a tiny dummy, specially designed for premature babies, which will help stimulate her ability to suck and swallow in preparation for feeding, and also provide her with comfort.

Touch Your premature baby's skin is incredibly sensitive to touch as she has more receptors in her skin than you do. Very light, "tickling" touch can be irritating to your baby, and she'll prefer a firm, gentle pressure that will help her feel secure. If your baby was born very prematurely, then her skin may be too sensitive to cope with lots of touching, which could overstimulate her. You can place one of your fingers in her hand for her to grasp, or very gently lay a hand or finger on her.

Touch is the first sense your baby develops, so she will know when she is being touched and can let you know if she finds the touch comforting or if it is irritating through a range of facial expressions and movements (see How your baby talks to you, p.52).

Your baby will also feel more comfortable and secure if she is surrounded and supported in the incubator, so nurses will often make a "nest" to go around her so she has something to push against, like being in the womb.

Taste Research has shown that babies prefer sweet tastes, even while they are still in the womb – a baby will swallow amniotic fluid faster if it is sweet.

Babies who are on neonatal units are often given a few drops of a sugar solution before a painful procedure, such as a heel-prick test or putting in a cannula, and this appears not only to distract them but also to actually reduce the pain (see p.60 for more on pain and your baby).

Smell Your premature baby is able to detect odours and will get to know your smell very quickly after birth. She'll be able to recognize you by your smell and it will help soothe her, especially as premature babies have their eyes shut for much of the time. Try putting a muslin or small teddy down your top so that it smells of you, then put it in the incubator with your baby to comfort her.

Your baby will also be able to smell very strong and overpowering odours, such as perfume and disinfectants, so try to avoid using anything that is likely to irritate her.

When you hold your baby close to you, she will begin to recognize the smell of your milk. This may make the process of breastfeeding easier when she is ready to start, as she'll already know what to expect and what she is searching for.

Crying Premature babies cry very little at first, and when they do it is often for only a short amount of time. They may be easily comforted by a touch or a few soft words. Smelling you or hearing your voice may be enough to settle them.

Movement Very premature babies have little muscle tone, which means their muscles are loose and floppy, so if they are left in an unsupported position, their limbs may splay out. Your baby will soon start to develop muscle tone as she grows older. You will see her move and flex her arms and legs, and even suck on her fingers. Before long, she'll be able to turn her head to look at you.

Twin comfort When they are stable, twins may spend some time in the same incubator or cot, which can be comforting for them.

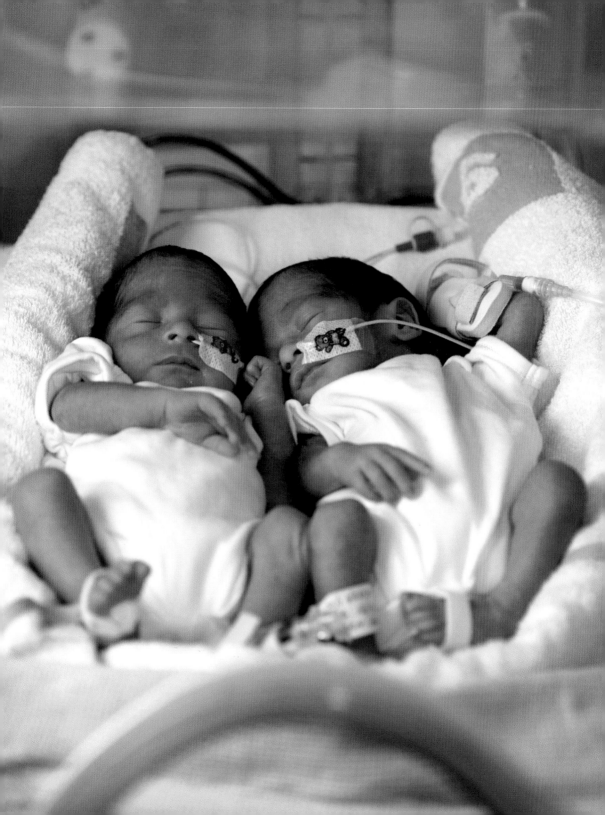

Bonding with your baby

When you see your tiny baby in an incubator, it may seem like bonding will be very hard. But he will communicate with you from his earliest days and, as you respond, you'll get to know each other and the bond will start to grow.

Bonding can be difficult when you feel anxious, and some parents are scared to get too attached to their baby in the very early days, especially if he is very small or sick, in case they lose him.

Try to think of it this way – those few precious moments when you might bond with your baby only to lose him can not be any worse than having lost your baby and not having started to connect with him. Even those few hours or days of memories are so special, and the regrets that parents are more likely to have if they have not formed any kind of relationship are much greater.

Watch out for moments when your baby is awake and alert as he may look at you or turn his head towards you when you talk to him. The beginning of this two-way communication is very special and is an exciting part of your growing relationship with your baby.

MY STORY

Dana says...

"**For the first couple of days I wanted him to die. It was horrible. I thought, let him just go, let him just go peacefully and not have any pain. I just didn't want him to be in pain.**

After a few days, where he seemed to be stable and he was still breathing, even though it was with a monitor, I looked at him and realized, 'He is my boy! How could I not want him? That's it, this boy is coming home.'

I said I'm never doing this again. I want two children – my girl and my boy. We just kept positive: lots of singing; we put our iPods in there and let him listen to nice music. We tried to do as much as we could, and we just fell in love with him, even though we couldn't hold him for a while. But once we did hold him, then that confirmed to me that, oh goodness, I love this child."

Dana, mum to Erin and Max

How your baby talks to you Even a very tiny, very premature baby can communicate with you, and you'll quickly get to know your own baby and what he likes and dislikes. As well as understanding what causes him stress, you'll see him relax when you soothe him, which is very rewarding and helps you to bond with him.

If your baby doesn't like something, he may:
- Pull his hand or foot away when it's touched
- Grimace
- Turn his head away
- Arch his body
- Frown
- Cry.

If he is stressed, he might also:
- Have hiccups
- Make jerky or flailing movements
- Startle more easily than usual
- Yawn
- Not sleep well
- Avoid eye contact
- Spread his fingers wide
- Extend his arms and legs.

> "You concentrate on his health rather than trying to bond. I had to put my faith in the medical team – the bonding came later."
>
> *Nick, dad to Xavier*

If your baby is relaxed, you may see:

- His breathing becoming regular
- His oxygen saturation settling
- His heart rate settling.

Even when sedated, babies can still react. If stressed, their oxygen consumption goes up, they can tense up, their breathing becomes erratic, and you can see that they're not comfortable at all. You can help decrease your baby's stress by:

- Being aware of how he reacts to light, sound, and touch and adjusting what you do accordingly

- Talking or singing to him; the sound of your familiar voice will comfort him
- Positioning him in the fetal position (on his tummy with knees tucked underneath him and bottom in the air).

The nurses who are looking after your baby will be constantly checking for any signs of distress, and if a baby seems to be behaving unusually – for instance, if a normally "feisty" baby is quieter than normal – they will bring this to the attention of the doctors caring for him.

In motion Your baby may tell you he is feeling stressed or unsettled by making jerky movements, and he may also startle more easily than usual.

Yawning Your baby may yawn if she's stressed or upset. However, she may just be telling you she's sleepy, and if she looks relaxed, she probably is. If you're worried, tell the nurse.

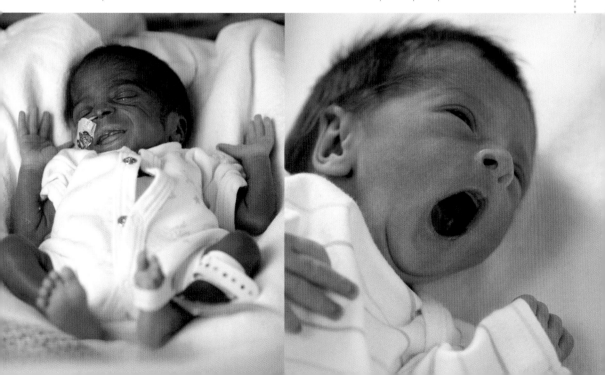

What can I do for my baby?

Whether it's holding her hand, talking and singing to her, or changing her nappy, there's a lot you can do for your baby while she's on the unit. The nurses will tell you what she's ready for and show you how to do it.

The nurses will encourage you to become as involved as possible in your baby's daily care. Don't worry about not knowing how to do things, or being all fingers and thumbs around your baby – the nurses will show you exactly how to handle her and care for her, including cleaning and nappy changing.

You may feel awkward sitting next to your baby's incubator if she is fast asleep, and worry that you're in the way or that you don't have a role to play among all the professionals on the unit who are caring for your baby. This couldn't be further from the truth, as even when your baby is sleeping you

"When he was in the incubator we would hold his hand or put our hands on his head. We would talk to him and read him stories."

Ross, dad to Freddie

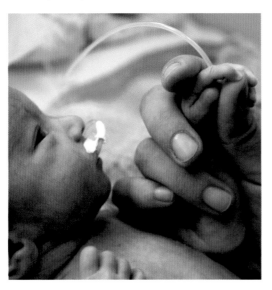

Holding hands A gentle, loving touch is a wonderful way to communicate with your baby, especially when she's not yet ready for cuddles.

are forming relationships with the nurses who are looking after her.

You can:

- Touch your baby (see p.58)
- Talk to your baby
- Read to your baby (it's never too early for this!)
- Sing to your baby
- Record voices for nurses to play to your baby when you're not there
- Bring things for your baby to look at – for instance, the staff can stick pictures of the family inside the cot
- Place small teddy bears inside your baby's incubator; these will have your scent so will give her comfort
- Express milk to be given to your baby when the time is right.

Becoming involved in your baby's practical care while on the unit can be a daunting prospect. You may feel out of your depth and want to leave the

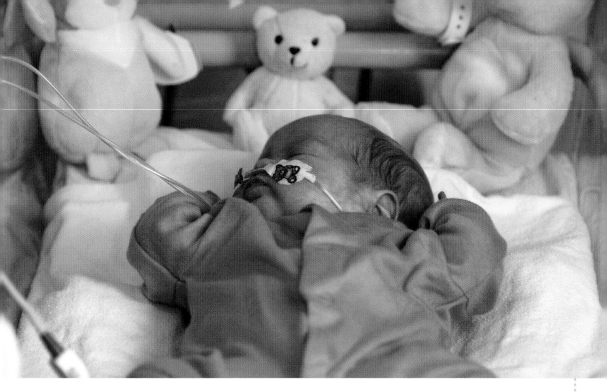

changing, bathing, and feeding to the staff. But it is helpful for both you and your baby if you become involved in her routine. There is lots of practical care you can carry out for your baby while she is on the unit, whether she is in an incubator and on a ventilator, or is "rooming in", preparing to go home. Depending on how small or sick your baby is you may be able to:

- Change her nappies
- Oil her skin
- Clean her face and eyes
- Bath her when she's stable enough
- Cuddle her – even babies on a ventilator can be cuddled once they are stable (see p.58).

She will know by the sound of your voice and your smell that you are caring for and handling her. This will reassure her and increase the bond between you. Some mums and dads are extremely nervous about handling their baby but the more they do it, the more practice they get, and the happier and more confident they become.

Cuddly company Soft toys or other items that smell of you will be comforting for your baby when you can't be with her.

Changing nappies

The nurses will show you how to clean your baby's bottom and how to change her nappy when she's stable enough for you to do it. Your baby will need to wear nappies that are specially designed for premature babies, as regular nappies will be too big.

You change a premature baby's nappy the same way you'd change any baby's nappy, except that if she's in an incubator, you'll be doing it through the portholes, which you might find intimidating at first. You'll soon become practiced though, and the nurses will always be on hand if you're unsure about anything.

There may be wires attached to your baby that you'll have to look out for, but the nurses will tell you which ones are important and mustn't be dislodged and which ones can be removed briefly.

while you're changing a nappy. Because your baby's skin is so delicate, you can't use baby wipes to clean her, because her skin will be too sensitive to the chemicals and they will irritate it. You'll need to use cotton wool and sterile water instead.

The nurses will show you exactly what to do and will stay with you.

Remember your baby's skin is very thin and fragile, so you'll need to wash her gently to avoid making her skin sore. Perfumed baby products are not suitable for your baby's delicate skin as

> **"The nurse said 'Are you ready to change a nappy?'**
> **I thought she was speaking to someone else.**
> **I said, 'Do you think I'm ready for it?'"**
>
> *Bal, dad to Leo*

Washing your baby When you wash your baby's face you need to use sterile water and gauze. If she has a tube in her nose or mouth, she may tend to get crusty lips, which can be difficult to clean.

Bathing your baby can be great for bonding and will be good practice for when you're ready to take her home. Very premature babies will just have their hands, face, and nappy area washed while they are inside the incubator, but older babies may be able to have a bath, which can be fun for both of you.

they can cause irritation. Sterile water will clean your baby just fine.

When you clean your baby's eyes, always use a fresh piece of gauze for each eye, just as you would for a term baby. Don't use cotton wool to clean your baby's eyes.

Freshen up One task you can undertake early on is to clean your baby's face with gauze and a little cooled, boiled water, even if she still has tubes in her mouth or nose.

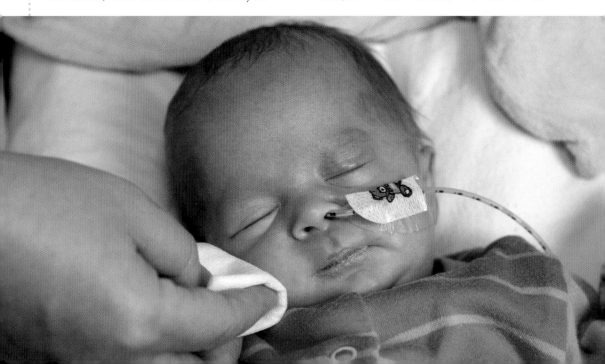

It's natural to be very tentative at first, but the nurses will show you how firm you can be and the position to hold her. It can be nerve-wracking caring for your baby, but you will get used to it.

Baby massage Babies on the neonatal unit often experience touch that hurts or is uncomfortable when they have tests and treatments. Massaging your baby is a wonderful way to counteract this with positive touch, and will also help you to relax. Massage could also help improve the development of your baby. Its advantages include:

- Building your confidence in caring for your baby
- Encouraging bonding and attachment
- Promoting breastfeeding
- Helping with postnatal depression.

As premature babies' skin is so fragile, not all babies may be at a suitable stage to be massaged, so check with the nurses first.

Once your baby is ready for massaging to begin, the nurses will guide you through what to do. They will use a doll to show you where and how to place your hands, and also the amount of pressure that should be applied. Premature babies find a light, sensitive touch tickly and irritating, so you will need to use a firm, but gentle approach. You will be able to practise the techniques on the doll if you feel unsure about what to do.

As well as being a lovely experience for you and your baby and a chance for you both to relax, massage is a great way for you to take part in her care when she is stable enough.

Time for you A really important thing you can do for your baby is to take time off. All parents need time for themselves, to get an emotional break as well as to do all the practical things that everyday life demands. The less stressed you are, the more you'll be able to enjoy your baby.

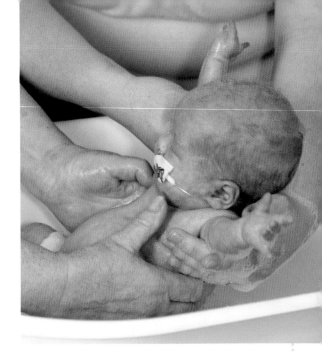

First bath The nurses will show you how to hold your baby safely and securely when you bath her. It may seem daunting at first, but you'll quickly get used to it.

TWINS AND TRIPLETS
Practical care

There isn't a formula for dividing your time between two or more babies. One baby may be healthier than the other, but they both need your attention. Trust your instincts and respond to their needs as you see fit.

Parents tend to get to know their babies quickly and will care for each of them in turn, so if they changed one baby's nappy last time, they'll change a different baby the next time.

Where possible, twins can share an incubator as it's good for them to be together. This won't usually happen while they still need help with their breathing as the incubator amplifies sound and two CPAP machines (see p.31) will make a lot of noise.

The power of touch

When your baby is stable enough, you'll be able to cuddle him against your chest. This skin-to-skin contact is brilliant for bonding and is also good for your baby's health and development.

Touch can be rewarding for both you and your baby. However, although it may seem instinctive to stroke a hand or a cheek lightly, he may not like this as his skin is so sensitive. Try a comfort hold by spreading your hand over his chest or holding his head in one hand and his feet or bottom in the other to create a sense of being firmly cradled (see p.61).

The more premature the baby, the more important it is to handle him as little as possible

popping your baby down the front of your shirt and cuddling him close. When you do this, he should settle, his pulse will slow, and he may need less oxygen.

Kangaroo care is great for bonding, and if you're breastfeeding it can increase your milk supply. You may need to wait until your baby is stable before attempting this type of care, but when he is ready, you can cuddle him even if he

> **"It was probably day four that I held Erin. She came off the ventilator and I just held her with tubes everywhere. It was the first time I realized she was mine."**
>
> *Dana, mum to Erin and Max*

until he is stable. This doesn't prevent you from touching him, but you may notice that when the doctors turn him over to examine him, or the nurses need to change his nappy, he becomes temporarily unsettled. Don't worry – he'll soon calm down.

If you can't cuddle your baby because he's too small, fragile, or sick, you can still hold his hand or cradle him in a comfort hold as well as talk to him. You will soon start to notice how he responds when you touch him and get to know exactly what he likes.

Kangaroo care Research has shown that babies who are well enough benefit from skin-to-skin contact, which is sometimes known as "kangaroo care". This consists of literally

still has tubes attached and is on CPAP (see p.31).

When you're both ready, the nurses will help position him against you. Some units will have a boob tube on hand (dads can also wear it) to help you hold your baby more securely, but you don't need anything other than your hands. If your baby has lots of tubes and wires, the nurses may tape them to you so they stay put.

Once your baby is ready for kangaroo care, it can be very rewarding. When your baby's care is mainly in the hands of the doctors and nurses on the unit, it is a very special way to bond with him that is exclusive to you as his parents.

First cuddles Holding your baby like this, against your body, is known as kangaroo care and you'll be able to do it even if she still has tubes attached.

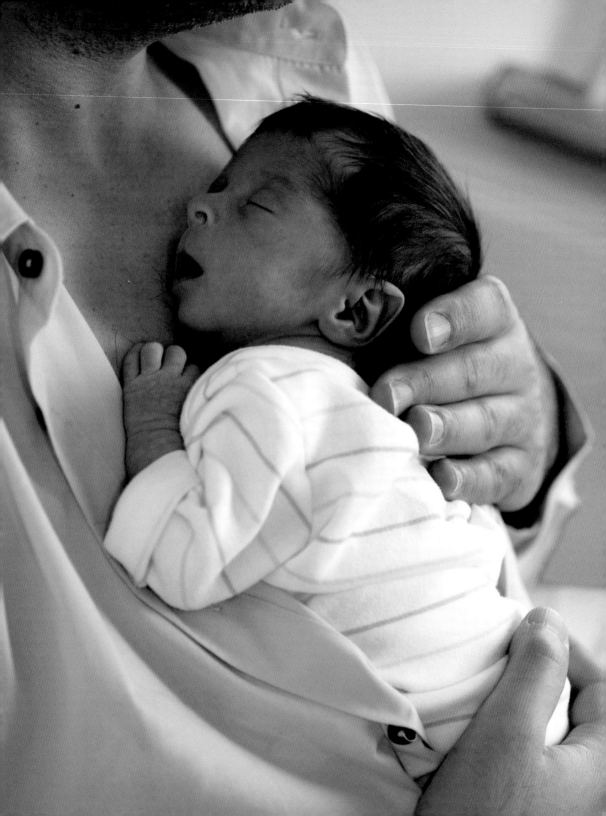

Keeping your baby comfortable

All parents dread the thought of their baby feeling pain or discomfort, but painful procedures are sometimes necessary. She'll have pain relief and you can help soothe her by touching and talking to her.

Is my baby in pain? There is no doubt that babies feel pain as shown by their altered behaviour and pulse rate when painful procedures are carried out. A premature baby may show pain by pulling away a hand or foot, squeezing her eyes shut, furrowing her brow, or screwing up her face. Her heart rate, blood pressure, skin tone, and oxygen saturation may also be affected.

For many years, neonatologists assumed that premature babies did not feel pain in the same way that older children do. This is clearly wrong and it is important for doctors to remember this whenever they carry out procedures. In many units, babies are given one or two drops of a sugar solution by mouth just before a blood test or putting in a cannula. This has been shown to work as well as a painkiller, and it takes effect very rapidly. You may notice that if your baby has just been given her sugar water she'll seem much more relaxed during a blood test.

When babies are on a ventilator, they have a constant infusion of morphine to sedate them and reduce any pain or anxiety they may feel. If a baby is on morphine, she won't need the sugar solution too.

If your baby was born very early you may notice a frightening number of tubes going into her veins, arteries, and umbilical vessels. The reason for this is that once they have been inserted they can be used for monitoring and thus minimize the number of painful blood tests that have to be done.

Sugar solution A few drops of sugar water given just before a procedure can provide quick and effective pain relief for your baby.

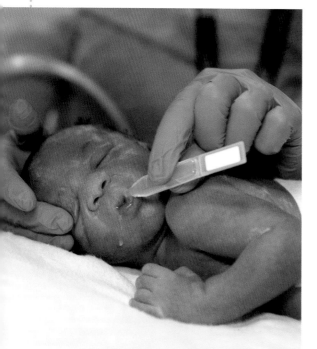

Your baby's position The more contained your baby is, the less stressed she feels and this helps with her physical development. She will be most comfortable on her front with her knees curled towards her chest and her arms close to her face with her hands free.

When the concept of treating babies in premature baby units was developed, doctors and nurses saw that babies did better if they were placed on their tummies to sleep. They required less oxygen, their breathing was less compromised, and they did better overall. It's important for them to be curled up with their feet under their tummies because it makes them feel secure and cocooned, just as they would be in the womb.

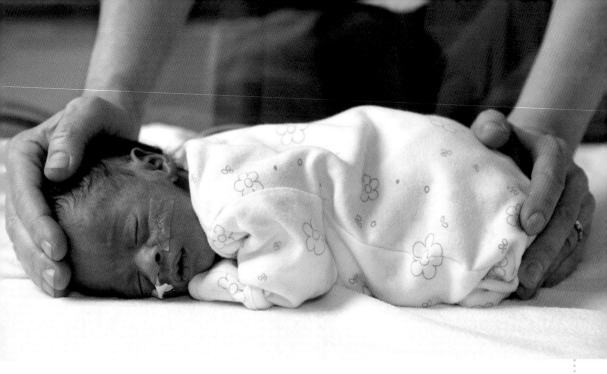

Because babies did better on their tummies on neonatal units, experts assumed that this would be better for them when they went home as well. So in the 1960s and 1970s, parents were told to put babies on their tummies to sleep and, as a result, the rate of cot death increased. It took until the 1980s for experts to recognize that there was a direct link between a baby's sleeping position and cot death.

Comfort hold Your baby will feel secure when you hold her gently but firmly in this way. Place one hand on her head and cradle her feet or bottom with the other.

goes home. This can be really difficult and she will cry at first. Being on her back, she's more likely to flail around and scare herself. One way to help her feel more secure on her back is to swaddle her,

> " Because he's had so much intervention, Leo gets cross and scared when people touch him. It is upsetting. "
> *Sophie, mum to Samuel and Leo*

Tiny babies in intensive care are closely monitored, so sleeping on their tummies is not a problem. They are attached to monitors that will tell the medical team if they stop breathing, if their heart rate changes, or if they need more oxygen. As soon as your baby is big enough and well enough, though, she will need to learn to sleep on her back and it's very important to get her used to this before she

although it's important that you use just one layer of a thin sheet, to avoid overheating.

Babies' heads are very mouldable during the first weeks and months, which means that they may develop flat sides to their heads. In order to prevent this, the incubator mattresses are very soft, the babies are turned frequently, and sometimes they are even given a tiny soft pillow.

Feeding your baby

It may be some time before your baby is able to feed from the breast or a bottle. He may not even be able to digest milk yet, in which case he will be given all the nutrients he needs via a vein.

How your baby is fed will depend on how early he was born and whether the doctors think he is ready to digest milk. Two terms you will hear if you're present during the ward rounds are "enteral" and "parenteral". Enteral means going into the stomach, while parenteral means going into a vein, and they

TPN is usually infused into a large vein, which means that the doctor has to insert a very fine, pliable tube, known as a long line, into a vein and feed it along until it is almost in the heart. Your baby then receives the nutrients directly into his bloodstream.

> "You express literally millilitres to begin with. Even if it was 1ml, the milk was put into syringes and then into the nasogastric tube."
>
> *Dana, mum to Erin and Max*

refer to the different ways your baby may be given nutrition on the unit. Once your baby is ready to be fed milk, whether this is given by tube feeding (either via the nose or mouth), bottle-feeding, or, eventually breastfeeding, you can be involved in providing him with essential nutrition. In fact, if you are able to express milk, then you will be providing your baby with the most important thing to help him grow stronger. If you are unable to express, then you will be able to be fully involved in feeding your baby special premature formula.

Total parenteral nutrition (TPN) If you have a very premature baby he will almost certainly need total parenteral nutrition. This is a fluid that is given directly into a vein and contains the correct combination of protein, carbohydrate, salts, and fat for your baby. The exact make up of the TPN is adjusted according to the results of blood tests and the age of the baby.

Unfortunately, like every procedure carried out in the unit, a long line does have potential problems, which mean that it may have to be removed earlier than planned and replaced with another one. The most common problems include blockage of the line and infection. Sometimes it is very difficult to thread a long line up a baby's vein and several attempts are needed.

The length of time your baby needs TPN depends on how early he was born and how ill he may be, but it is usually given for between several days and several weeks after birth. Because of the potential problems with having a long line for TPN, babies are kept on this form of feeding only for as long as they absolutely need it.

As soon as your baby is ready, and this is often at the same time as starting TPN, he can be weaned onto milk. This needs to be given via a nasogastric or orogastric tube, inserted respectively through the nose or mouth (see opposite).

Nasogastric/orogastric feeds Before your baby can suck in a coordinated way, he can still be fed milk (enteral feeds) as long as he is well enough to be able to digest it. By far the best milk for your baby is your own breast milk. If you cannot express your own milk, then your baby may receive donated breast milk (see p.65). Breast milk is easier to digest than formula milk, contains antibodies that help protect your baby from infection, and contains the right amount of protein, carbohydrate, and fat for him to flourish. Babies who are fed expressed breast milk are also less likely to have complications such as necrotizing enterocolitis (NEC) (see p.79).

A tiny flexible tube is inserted into the baby's nose or mouth and gently pushed until it reaches the stomach, and the tube is taped beside your baby's mouth to keep it secure. This is a painless procedure that shouldn't bother your baby. The nurses test that it is in the right place using litmus paper to check for acidity (the stomach contents are acidic); then they attach a syringe and slowly pour milk into it, allowing gravity to carry the milk down the tube into the stomach.

The nurses usually start by giving small quantities of milk every few hours and slowly build up the amount of milk over the next few days, if your baby seems to be tolerating and digesting the milk. If your baby vomits a significant amount of milk or if there is milk left in the stomach before the next feed is due, it may be that your baby is not digesting the milk properly. This will be checked by gently suctioning out any remaining stomach contents. If undigested milk is found, the nurses may decide to give your baby smaller quantities of milk more slowly – or even to give small amounts of milk continuously so that the stomach never contains more than a tiny amount of milk. Your baby may be fed via a nasogastric or orogastric tube for as long as he needs, until he is stronger and able to move onto bottle-feeding or breastfeeding.

The nurses may teach you how to help them with the feeds, for example, by showing you how to

Tube feeds Even before your baby is able to suck, if he's ready to digest milk he can have it through a tube that goes into his tummy via his nose or mouth.

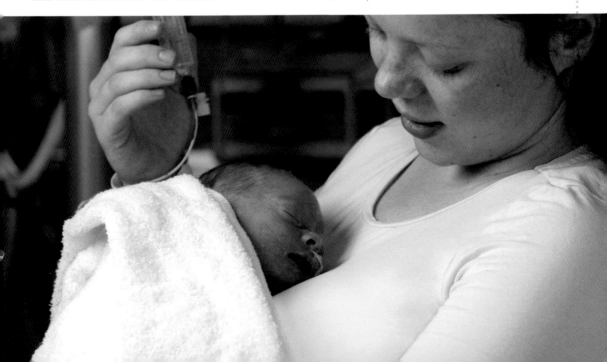

hold your baby and the syringe and tube. They may also recommend offering your baby a dummy while he is fed so that he understands the link between sucking and being fed and also practises sucking, so when he is ready for bottle-feeding or breastfeeding, the motion won't be too difficult.

When will my baby start having milk?

Before TPN is started in newborns, all they will have had is a drip containing water and glucose, but no actual nutrition. This is similar to what breastfed term babies will experience, as they will only have colostrum for the first few days. This means that the doctors have a little while to decide whether to give TPN or milk feeds.

Giving a tiny bit of milk to a baby, however small, is thought to be a good thing in one way as it primes his gut and gets it working. However, a problem that can affect very premature, small-for-dates, or very

unwell babies is inflammation of the gut, called necrotizing enterocolitis (NEC) (see p.79), which is possibly sometimes related to early formula milk feeds. Although rare, NEC is potentially serious.

On other hand, putting in a long line for TPN does carry risks, including infection, leakage, and blockage of the line.

So the medical team will make the decision for each individual baby about what they feel is best. If your baby is particularly vulnerable and thought to be at higher risk of developing NEC, it's likely that he will have TPN for the first five days at least before slowly trying milk feeds.

Types of milk Breast milk is the number one choice for all babies but even more so if they are premature. Even if your premature baby is unable to feed from either breast or bottle, your expressed breast milk can still be given to him through his

Expressing milk If you express your breast milk at least every four hours around the clock, you will have a greater chance of producing enough for your baby.

Storing your milk Expressed milk needs to be kept in a fridge or freezer in the unit, ready for you or the staff to give it to your baby.

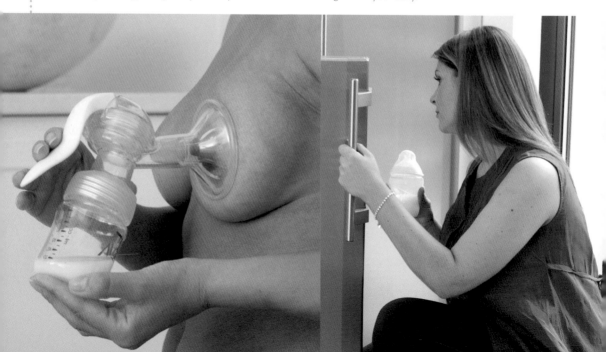

nasogastric tube. The milk of a mother who has given birth prematurely is different from that of the mother of a term baby, and is particularly well suited to the nutritional needs of her baby.

Some very vulnerable babies will be given donor breast milk if the mother is unable to express her

and don't get too discouraged. There is a knack to expressing so don't hesitate to ask for as much support as you need. Being near your baby may help the flow of milk, and the nurses can put screens around his cot or incubator to give you some privacy.

> " My milk came in quite quickly and I expressed tons and donated a lot to the milk bank. I was really lucky with my milk because a lot of women can't do it. "
>
> Dana, mum to Erin and Max

own milk. This is milk that has been expressed by another mother and then pasteurized to make it safe to give to other babies. Only a few babies will have donated breast milk as the process of pasteurization removes some of the beneficial properties that your own breast milk would have. Therefore, generally, if your baby is not having your breast milk, he will have the specifically designed pre-term formula.

Expressing milk It is best to start expressing breast milk, if you are able to, as soon as possible after your baby is born. Ideally, you should be expressing every three to four hours, both day and night. The more you express your milk, the more you will make. The reverse is also true: the less milk that you express, the smaller the amount of milk that will be produced.

The nurses on the unit will show you how to express milk manually or with a pump – either a hand pump or an electric pump. On the first day, the recommendation is that hand expressing is generally best; but afterwards, use whatever method you feel happiest with.

It can be difficult to express milk to begin with, especially as you're going through a very stressful time, so try to relax when you do it

Breast milk needs to be stored in the fridge or freezer. It will keep in the fridge for three to five days or in the freezer for three months.

Donating milk There are a number of milk banks around the country that take breast milk if you have more than your baby needs and you would like to be a donor. There will be some paperwork to complete to see if you are a suitable donor, and

TIPS
Expressing milk

- Sit near your baby when you're expressing, as this will encourage the flow of breast milk.
- If your baby isn't with you, hearing other babies cry can sometimes help with your "let-down" reflex, which triggers the release of milk from your breasts.
- Having a shower can help start the let-down reflex.
- Try using fenugreek, a herbal remedy that can help to get your milk production going (seek medical advice before taking anything you're unsure about).
- If all else fails, ask your GP to prescribe domperidone, a drug that works to stimulate the production of a hormone that helps you produce breast milk.

you'll need to be tested for HIV, along with hepatitis B and C . The doctors on the unit should be able to do the blood test for you. Generally, the expressed milk can be collected from the unit or from your home, whichever is more convenient. You won't be paid for your donation, but you'll feel rewarded knowing you're helping another premature baby.

Moving on The decision when to stop tube feeding a baby, and begin him on breastfeeding or bottle-feeding will be different for each baby. The staff on the unit will not stop tube feeding until your baby is able to coordinate sucking and swallowing. Your baby's sucking skills are not completely developed, so getting him to feed from the breast or bottle will require plenty of practice and patience.

The staff will show you the correct position for holding your baby and how to encourage him to latch on properly during breastfeeding. As with term babies, it is important that your baby takes all of the nipple and the areola (area around the nipple) in his mouth, otherwise he will have to work harder to get milk. Sucking is tiring for your baby, and he will have to make the connection between sucking, breathing, and swallowing.

Your baby may not take in much milk when he first starts breastfeeding, and may only attempt it once or twice a day. Don't rush him – he'll get better with practice and will soon be feeding every few hours.

If your baby is unable to suck for very long, then he will receive his remaining feed through a tube. Carry on with expressing though, as your milk can be stored, ready to use for bottle-feeding.

> "It was difficult expressing when I wasn't with him but I kept going for seven and a half months. I felt it was something I could do for him."
>
> *Claudia, mum to Chase*

Breastfeeding You may already find that during kangaroo care your baby smells your milk and seeks your breast. He is probably unable to latch on at this stage and only nuzzles or licks for a short time before falling asleep. This is good practice for your baby to understand where his milk comes from when he is strong enough.

The staff on the unit will look for signs that your baby is ready to start breastfeeding, and will guide and support you and your baby through the first and subsequent attempts. One indication that your baby is ready for breastfeeding is if he turns his head and opens his mouth wide in search of food when his cheek is stroked. This reaction is an instinctive behaviour known as the rooting reflex.

Bottle-feeding If you are able to express enough milk, then your baby can also be bottle-fed. This means your baby will still be receiving your milk even when you're not there, and also allows dad to be involved in the feeding process.

On some units, your baby may be offered cup feeding as an alternative to bottle-feeding. In theory this is a good way of transitioning from tube to breast without using bottles. It means that your baby will only be sucking from the breast and not be confused by sucking from the bottle.

If your baby has been using a dummy, or has been breastfeeding, then he will already have practice when introduced to bottle-feeding. The bottle teats used for premature babies are smaller and softer than those used for term babies because premature babies are smaller and have weaker muscles. As your baby becomes stronger, the size of the bottle teat will change.

The nurses will show you how to feed your baby and wind him. They will show you how to hold him correctly, and how to watch to check that he is sucking properly. Babies tend to swallow more air during bottle-feeding than during breastfeeding, causing them to feel uncomfortable. It is important that the milk in the bottle fills the teat and neck, to help reduce the amount of air your baby swallows.

Before you take your baby home, the staff will make sure you know how to make up feeds and wash and sterilize feeding equipment. If there's anything you're unsure of, ask as many times as you need to.

Wee and poo If your baby is dehydrated, he will have fewer wet nappies than usual. When newborn babies are first in the neonatal unit, the doctors and nurses watch them very closely to work out how many millilitres per kilogram of body weight of urine they are passing per hour. The nappies are weighed to check exact quantities of liquid – each millilitre of urine weighs one gram – and every millilitre makes a difference when babies are so tiny. If a baby needs to be given extra fluids, these calculations are critical. The other thing to watch out for is dark brown wee, which can be a sign of liver problems in a baby.

Premature babies may not pass their first poo very quickly as they've had nothing by mouth. When they do poo, though, it will be meconium, a sticky, tarry green-black substance that has built up in your baby's gut in the womb. Sometimes, if babies take a long time to poo, doctors might use a glycerine chip (a tiny suppository) to help things along, as in such small babies it can be hard to get everything working.

Once your baby has passed meconium, his poo will change to normal newborn poos that may be

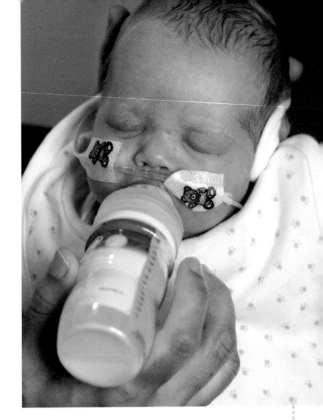

Bottle-feeding Whether you are giving your baby expressed breast milk or the special premature baby milk formula, she will be receiving all the nutrients she needs.

liquid or semi-solid and might be yellow, orange, or brown. This will happen whether he is being fed enterally (via the stomach) or parenterally (via a vein). There are a few poo colours that doctors look out for and worry about:

● White liquid: This means that the baby is just passing milk straight through his body without it being processed properly.

● Red: If there is blood in your baby's poo, this is a sign that there is inflammation in his gut.

● Putty-coloured: pale poo can indicate a problem with the way the liver handles certain waste products in the body.

If your baby has any of these, the medical team will investigate and decide on the best treatment.

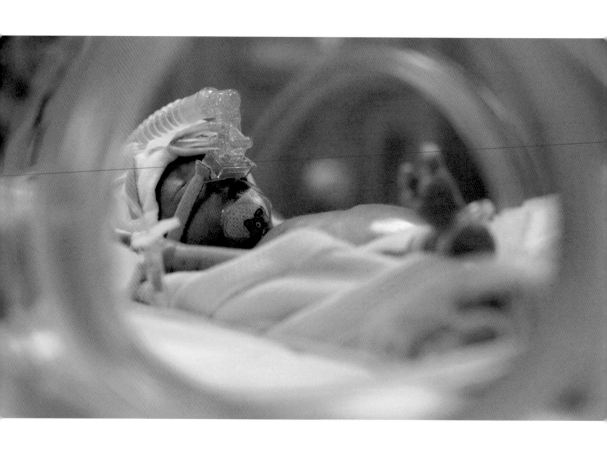

Monitoring
& treatment

An array of devices attached to your baby constantly monitor her well-being, and enable her treatment to be adjusted as necessary to meet her needs.

Monitoring your baby

Your baby will have been carefully monitored at antenatal checks throughout your pregnancy and, once she is born, this monitoring will continue on the neonatal unit to assess her well-being and development.

When you walk into a neonatal unit you will face what can be a daunting number of machines, and you will hear monitors going off frequently, with a siren-like sound. You will get used to them in time, but it can be a scary experience at first.

The point of those monitors is to indicate when a baby's heart rate is too fast or too slow, or to draw attention to oxygen levels dropping, or changes in the baby's temperature or blood pressure. The doctors and nurses are checking the babies constantly, and the monitors will alert them to any changes so that they can adjust the baby's treatment and respond rapidly to her needs.

The monitoring is set up to reduce any stress or upset felt by the babies as much as possible. Monitors are attached to your baby to give a constant reading without the need to prod or poke her all the time. However, as soon as monitoring involves pricking your baby with a needle, which is necessary to obtain blood for testing, then it may become painful. Giving a few drops of sugar water will help. Babies seem to love it – it helps to distract them and relieves the pain of the needle.

Tubes and needles You'll often see doctors taking blood from a baby's heel, called a heel-prick test. Premature babies have fragile skin, so when a heel-prick blood test is carried out, there needs

Inserting a cannula A small tube called a cannula is being inserted into a vein. It can be used to take blood samples for testing as well as to give drugs and fluids to your baby.

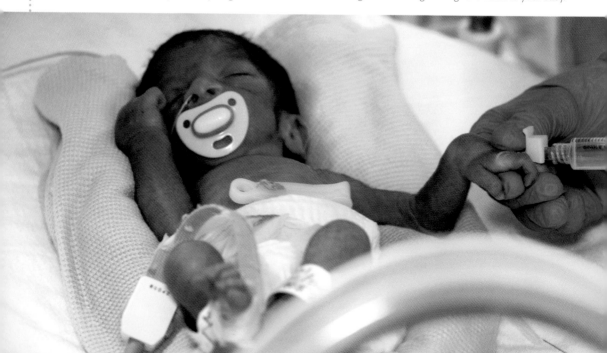

to be a good blood supply to the heel, so doctors don't have to squeeze too hard to get the blood out.

Sometimes a baby needs a cannula, which is a little needle with a silastic (silicone rubber) tube over it. Once the cannula is in, the needle is taken out and the tube is left in place. The cannula can first be used to take blood, and then it will be attached to a drip so that the baby can be given fluids or medication.

A longer flexible tube is sometimes referred to as a catheter – for instance, doctors will refer to an umbilical artery catheter. A very premature baby who needs a lot of monitoring will generally have an umbilical artery catheter, if possible. This is inserted into one of the arteries in the umbilical cord and can be used for taking blood samples and monitoring the baby's blood pressure. A baby may also have a catheter inserted into the umbilical vein, which can be used to give drugs and fluids. As the umbilical cord doesn't have any nerves, inserting an umbilical catheter doesn't hurt.

Blood tests
Blood can be collected from your baby into little bottles and sent to the laboratory for testing, or it can be collected into fine tubes and tested immediately using machines in the unit.

The problem with testing blood is that tiny babies don't reproduce it quickly enough to replace what has been taken. For this reason, if a baby is very sick the doctors will log exactly how much blood they've taken each time, even if it's just 1ml. Once a certain amount of blood has been taken the baby will need a little top-up transfusion.

Blood gases It's important to have accurate readings of oxygen and carbon dioxide levels in your baby's blood as this helps the staff to assess whether your baby needs more help with breathing.

Full blood count This is to check the level of haemoglobin, which carries oxygen around the body; white blood cells, which are produced to fight infection; and platelets, which help the blood clot.

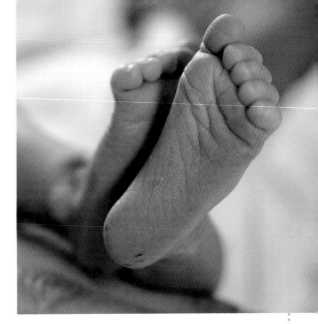

Heel-prick test Doctors and nurses will often take blood by pricking a baby's heel, and you may notice the little marks on your baby's feet where this has been done.

C-reactive protein (CRP) If the CRP is raised, there may be an infection, although this test doesn't indicate what the cause is.

Blood cultures If doctors suspect an infection, blood cultures are done to look for specific bacteria.

Urea and electrolytes Measuring these chemicals indicates how well the kidneys are functioning, and shows the levels of salt and potassium in the body.

Liver function tests (LFTs) This group of tests measure how the baby's liver is working.

Bilirubin This is a by-product of the breakdown of blood cells by the liver, and an excess can cause jaundice. Blood levels of bilirubin may be measured to determine the severity of jaundice.

Bone chemistry tests These measure calcium, phosphate, and alkaline phosphatase, which are all very important in bone growth.

Blood glucose This test measures the amount of sugar in your baby's blood. Very sick babies may have a high glucose level and may need to be given insulin for a short time.

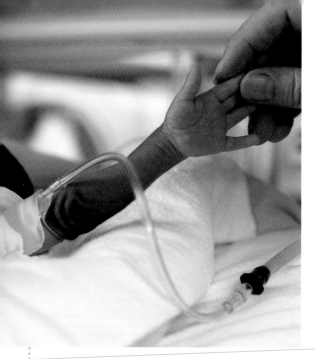

Checking blood pressure A premature baby's blood pressure is most commonly checked using a small cuff placed around the upper arm (as here) or leg.

Blood pressure

A baby's blood pressure is checked regularly to make sure it does not drop to too low a level. Low blood pressure means that blood is not circulating at the correct rate, so organs are not receiving enough oxygen and nutrients to function properly.

There are two ways of monitoring your baby's blood pressure. One is with a transducer, an electronic device attached to a line going into an artery that constantly monitors your baby's blood pressure. The other way is with a little cuff that goes around an arm or a leg and is inflated to give a measurement. A cuff can be used even on very tiny premature babies.

Oxygen saturation

The clip that goes on your baby's finger, hand, or foot shows what percentage of oxygen is going round her blood. It works by shining a light through the finger. It's used for adults as well.

Breathing

To measure your baby's respiratory rate, a sensor is placed on her to see how fast she is breathing in and out. The best place for this sensor is actually on the abdomen as babies move their abdomen much more than they move their chest when they breathe.

Cranial ultrasound

Newborn babies have a soft spot on the head, called a fontanelle. This is the perfect window into the brain through which doctors can perform an ultrasound scan. Ultrasound can give a lot of information about the baby's brain, including whether there has been a haemorrhage (bleeding) or if there is too much fluid in the brain.

Babies on the unit often wear little hats with a flap that can be undone so a doctor can easily do a scan without moving them. Cranial ultrasound isn't painful, though sometimes babies wriggle a little and the doctor will have to try to hold their heads still.

Eye tests

Babies who are born very early are given their first eye test when they reach around 32 weeks corrected gestational age (see p.116). This test is to check for retinopathy of prematurity (ROP), in which new little blood vessels develop when they shouldn't. In severe cases, this can lead to retinal detachment and blindness.

After this, the baby will be tested regularly to look for signs of ROP, or to monitor it and carry out laser treatment to destroy the abnormal blood vessels, if necessary. ROP is not common but the risk increases when babies have a lot of oxygen, so oxygen saturation levels are monitored carefully.

Hearing checks

All newborn babies in the UK have a hearing test before leaving hospital. This involves quiet clicking sounds being played into your baby's ear via a soft earpiece or through headphones and monitoring her responses. Premature babies will have this test before they leave the unit, and those who come into a high-risk category – for instance, if they've had meningitis or severe jaundice – will have further assessments.

Checking for hernias
A hernia occurs when there is a gap in the muscle wall of the abdomen. This allows the bowel to push through, making a bump that you can see through the skin. There are two common types of hernia: umbilical hernias, which appear in the umbilical region, and inguinal hernias, which appear in the groin. Premature babies are more likely to have a hernia than babies born at term, and doctors will check for them.

Umbilical hernia This is due to the gap left in the muscle wall where the umbilical vein and arteries were situated during pregnancy and just after birth. Usually the gap will close soon after birth, and in almost all babies, it will close by the age of a year.

Eye test All very premature babies on the unit will have regular eye tests to check for retinopathy of prematurity (ROP), which can cause long-term problems with sight.

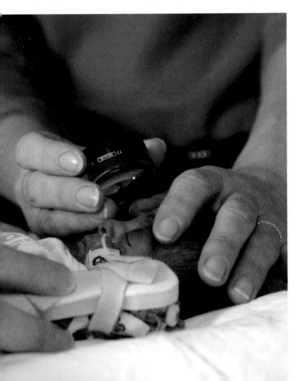

An operation is only rarely needed. Umbilical hernias occur in both girls and boys and are more common in some racial groups.

Inguinal hernia This type of hernia is more likely to occur in boys and is potentially more serious than umbilical hernia. In boys, it occurs due to the hole left in the muscle wall by the passage of the testes as they descend from the abdomen to the scrotum before birth. Rarely, girls can develop a weakness in the muscle wall in the groin area.

If your baby has an inguinal hernia, you will see a large swelling in the scrotum. Inguinal hernias can suddenly appear in the early weeks or months and need to be assessed by a doctor urgently.

Checking the hernia may be painful for your baby and crying will make it worse, so the doctor will try to relax him and will give pain relief. The doctor will then lie your baby on his back and try to gently ease the lump back into the abdomen. This will usually be possible, but most inguinal hernias will need an operation to close them as otherwise there is a risk of the bowel becoming stuck in the scrotum. The operation will usually be done at a specialist centre and will close the gap in the muscle permanently. It will be done under general anaesthetic and the baby will be left with a scar that is barely visible.

Consenting to procedures
Doctors and nurses will explain your baby's needs to you and will usually assume your consent to everyday procedures such as taking blood, inserting cannulas, and putting your baby on the ventilator.

If your baby needs an operation, the surgeon who will perform it will explain it to you and make sure you are aware of all the risks. You will need to sign a formal consent form for this. It is good practice for the hospital to request consent from parents for blood transfusions and exchange blood transfusions, although most units do not require you to sign a consent form for these procedures.

Treating your baby

If your baby needs treatment, the medical team will explain what this entails, and will talk to you about any potential side effects. If you have any questions, don't hesitate to ask the doctors or nurses.

The treatment your baby is offered and why it is necessary will always be explained to you. The amount of detail given to you will vary from doctor to doctor, so if you want more information or if you feel that the benefits or risks of a treatment haven't been fully explained, do ask. Sometimes life-saving treatments must be carried out immediately and there may be no time to explain in detail. Your baby may need to be ventilated or have CPAP (see p.31), or may develop a problem that requires urgent treatment in the unit or at a different hospital.

Medicines Babies on the neonatal unit will have all sorts of medication, depending on their needs. Painkillers are very important and are used a lot depending on what treatment the baby requires.

Babies on ventilators will usually be given morphine in the form of a continuous infusion. This means that they are not very aware of what's going on, and they also won't have any memory of what's happened afterwards – it's a "chilling-out" drug. If a baby has been on a ventilator for a long time, the medical team will wean him off the morphine rather than just stop it suddenly. Babies on the unit will be given other pain relief, too, including paracetamol and sugar solution (see p.60).

Other medication used on the unit includes antibiotics, drugs called inotropes, which increase

Phototherapy If your baby has jaundice, he'll be given this safe, effective treatment, which involves exposing him to a special light. His eyes are protected during the treatment.

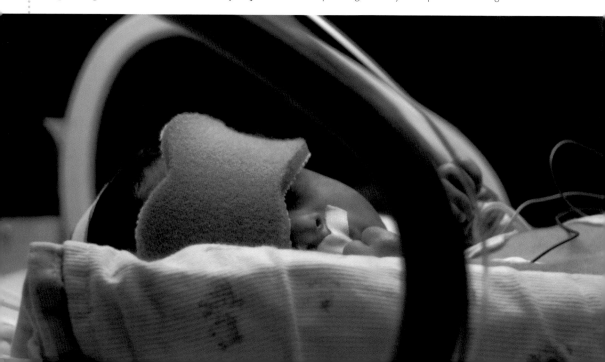

a baby's blood pressure, diuretics to help the baby pass more urine, vitamins, iron, phosphate, and steroids. If your baby is still having medication when you take him home, the nurses will go through everything very carefully with you so you know exactly what to do.

Jaundice This condition is very common in premature babies. It occurs when a baby's immature liver is unable to efficiently excrete bilirubin, a by-product of the breakdown of red blood cells, so levels build up in the blood.

It is quite easy for doctors to diagnose jaundice as the baby's skin will start to turn yellow a few days

Perspex box over his head. Phototherapy can be done from all sides and there are even special phototherapy mattresses and blankets.

When a baby is having phototherapy, the medical team is constantly trying to get a balance between the baby's need to be fed and cared for and his need to spend a lot of time under the lights. He will be stripped down to his nappy, because it's important to have as much of his body exposed to the light as possible. Babies having phototherapy may have diarrhoea and can also be a bit drowsy.

If your baby is jaundiced, he'll also be given lots of fluids to help flush bilirubin out of his system.

"We found that our baby had good days and bad days, and it was really hard to know what to expect."

Claudia, mum to Chase

after birth. When doctors notice that your baby has jaundice, they rarely worry, as phototherapy (see below) is given and is an effective way to keep the bilirubin levels low. The earlier a baby was born, the more readily doctors or nurses will start phototherapy because high bilirubin levels are potentially more damaging to very premature babies, especially in the early days.

If a baby becomes extremely jaundiced he is in danger of getting a condition called kernicterus, in which high levels of bilirubin cause brain damage. This is very rare, largely because procedures to deal with jaundice prevent it from happening.

Phototherapy If your baby has jaundice, the first thing the medical team will do is give him phototherapy. This is a very safe treatment that involves exposing him to a light that is similar to ultraviolet. Your baby's eyes need to be covered up, either with eye pads or by placing a little tinted

Exchange transfusions If the bilirubin levels aren't coming down with phototherapy, your baby might need an exchange transfusion, which means gradually replacing all your baby's blood with new blood, bit by bit. This can be done via umbilical lines – there are two arteries and a vein, so the old blood can be taken out of an artery and the new blood can go into the vein. Umbilical catheters can only be put in during the first days of life, as the cord dries up after this, but once in they can stay in place for as long as they are needed.

Blood incompatibilities The most common reason for an exchange transfusion is blood incompatibility. If you're rhesus negative, and you have a baby who is rhesus positive, you'll be given an injection (called anti-D) to try to stop you developing antibodies in your blood, so if you have another baby, he won't be affected. Without anti-D, your next baby could get antibodies that cross through the placenta from your blood into his blood. This can cause his blood to break down (haemolyze), leading to severe anaemia and jaundice. In extreme cases you might miscarry, but more commonly the baby will be born and quickly become very pale and jaundiced.

Rhesus incompatibility problems are generally solved by giving anti-D. However, sometimes ABO incompatibility can occur. This is an incompatibility between blood groups A, B, and O. It can be treated with phototherapy, and only very rarely is exchange transfusion needed. The outcome is excellent.

Babies coming into the unit from outside the hospital

If your baby has a problem that needs surgery or treatment the neonatal unit can't provide, he will need to be transferred out of the unit to another hospital.

worried about meeting completely new staff and about whether your baby will receive the same quality of care. This is very natural, but don't worry – your baby won't be transferred unless the staff are confident that he is ready.

If you've taken your newborn home and he then develops a problem that needs hospital treatment, such as jaundice or group B strep (a potentially serious infection that can develop in the first few days of life), he won't go back into the neonatal unit. Instead, he'll go to the children's ward or children's intensive care, even if he's only just gone home.

Cooling treatment

If a baby born after 36 weeks has had a very difficult time before or during the birth and his brain has been deprived of oxygen, he may benefit from cooling treatment. Research has shown that cooling slows down the

" He's had treatment in other hospitals; a double hernia repair, laser eye surgery... You name it, he's had it. "

Claudia, mum to Chase

Examples of this would be if the baby has a major heart problem, or a blocked or twisted bowel. If he does need to go to a different hospital, he will be transferred by the neonatal transport service (see p.25). After treatment or surgery, your baby may return to the neonatal unit he was transferred from. When he arrives back, skin swabs will be sent to the lab to look for bacteria and he will be nursed in an incubator. Doctors and nurses will wear gloves and aprons until the results of swabs come back clear. A baby who is born prematurely at home will be treated in a similar way in order to avoid bringing bacteria into the unit which could spread between babies.

If your baby is being transferred from a more intensive unit in another hospital, you may be

baby's metabolic rate and may prevent or reduce brain damage, depending on how severely affected he has been. The brain cells that have been starved of oxygen do not die straight away when kept at a cooler temperature.

Babies who undergo this treatment are placed on a special cooling mattress. The cooling is usually continued for 72 hours and the baby is then gradually re-warmed. To be beneficial the treatment needs to be started within six hours of birth.

Cooling treatment is only performed at specialist centres and isn't suitable for very premature babies.

Comforting cuddles If your baby is well enough to be held, cuddling can help soothe him. If not, just having you close by will be reassuring.

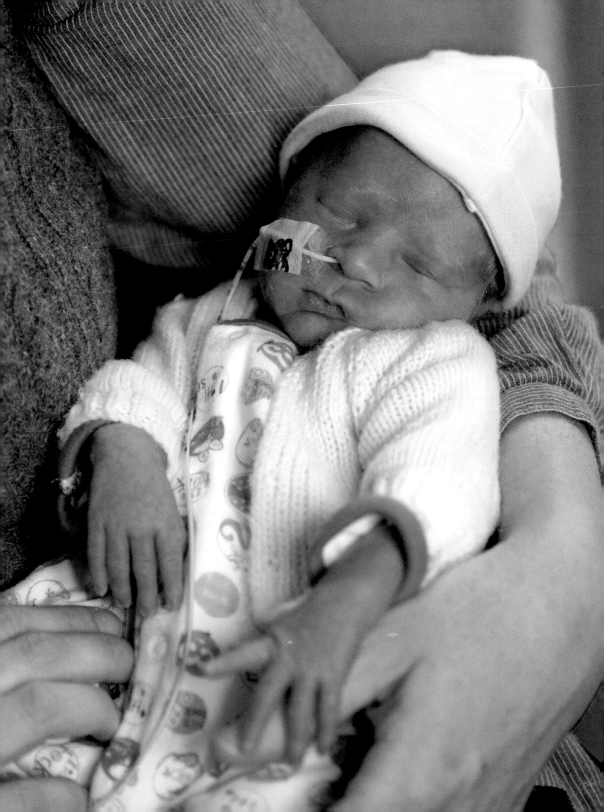

Complications of treatments

Any treatment your baby receives on the unit will be given because the benefits outweigh the risks. Unfortunately, sometimes treatments themselves can cause problems and the medical team is vigilant in checking for these.

All treatments offered to babies carry the risk of side effects or complications. This is because nothing can replace the womb in terms of the support a baby needs in order to grow and develop. You must trust the doctors and nurses to carry out the best care possible for your baby. If treatment is needed urgently, they may or may not have a chance to go through any possible side effects such as the ones listed below. Be sure to ask if you have any concerns or questions.

Pneumothorax This means that a tiny hole in the lung causes air to leak out of it. The air is then trapped in the space outside the lung causing the lung to collapse. This can happen at any time, even if a baby has not needed resuscitation, but is far more likely to occur if a baby is having CPAP (see p.31) or is being ventilated.

A pneumothorax can be relatively insignificant and cause no major problems; on the other hand, it can happen quickly, resulting in rapid deterioration of the baby and requiring urgent treatment.

Intraventricular haemorrhage One of the things parents most commonly worry about is their baby's brain. Being born early can result in a haemorrhage (bleeding) in the brain as the thin layer of cells lining the baby's ventricles (fluid-filled spaces in the brain) is more susceptible to damage.

The more premature a baby is, and the more unstable she is in the first week or so of life, the higher the chance of a haemorrhage occurring. The ventricles can easily be seen on an ultrasound scan through the soft spot (fontanelle). The extent of the haemorrhage tells doctors whether it is something they should be worried about and, in particular, whether there are likely to be any long-term problems for the baby's development. There are four grades of intraventricular haemorrhage, increasing in seriousness. Grade 1 is very minor, whereas grade 4 means there is bleeding into the brain itself.

The greater the extent of the haemorrhage, the greater the likelihood of long-term problems. A grade 1 haemorrhage carries no increased risk of long-term brain damage. If your baby has a grade 4 haemorrhage, particularly if it involves both sides of the brain, the doctors and nurses will be very worried that your baby is likely to suffer major long-term problems. These may mean difficulty with motor skills, such as walking, as well as problems with language or understanding.

Chronic lung disease If a baby still requires extra oxygen by the corrected gestational age of 36 weeks, she has chronic lung disease. This occurs in some babies as a direct result of the extra support they have needed with their breathing and is common in babies born very early. Some babies may still be on the ventilator, some will need CPAP either continuously or intermittently, while others breathe with no artificial support but require extra oxygen.

Gradually, as your baby gets better, the hope is that she will need less oxygen and less support with her breathing. It is usually just a matter of patience. Some babies are completely ready for home except that they still need extra oxygen. If the staff are

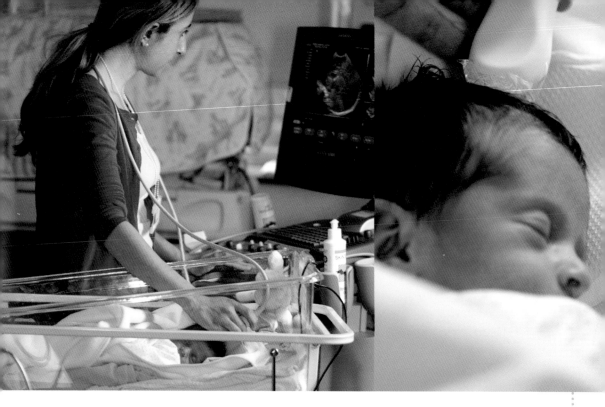

confident that you are able to provide all necessary care at home and expect that she will need extra oxygen for some time to come, they will discuss arranging oxygen for your home.

Ultrasound scan Doctors regularly use a portable scanner to check for signs of bleeding in a baby's brain. This can be done without moving the baby.

Sepsis (infection)

Premature babies are more susceptible to infection than babies born at term and the risk is increased because they have lines inserted into their bodies and solutions infused through these lines. Although great care is taken on all units to reduce the risk of infection, when a baby becomes unwell for whatever reason, the medical team usually assume that infection is a possible cause and will treat her with antibiotics.

Blood, urine, and sometimes samples of cerebrospinal fluid (CSF) are sent to the laboratory for testing to determine if infection is present. When the results are back, doctors know whether or not they need to continue giving antibiotics. Results normally take around 48 hours to come back as this is how long it takes for bacteria to grow. If no bacteria grow, it is unlikely that the baby has a serious infection.

Necrotizing enterocolitis (NEC)

Sometimes a baby can suddenly seem unwell – her tummy becomes tender and swollen, and she vomits or passes blood in her poo. These are all possible signs of NEC, which is severe inflammation of the bowel and can be fatal. Its exact cause is unknown, but it is more common in babies who are small for dates, very premature, or very unwell.

Doctors will usually arrange an X-ray, stop milk feeds, and start antibiotics. If the baby is very unwell, the medical team may need to put her on a ventilator, and an operation might be necessary.

Difficult decisions

Sometimes, despite the best efforts of the medical team, a baby's condition deteriorates and the outlook is poor. This does not mean that the baby will inevitably die, but the team will be honest with you about their concerns.

If a baby is so sick that the staff feel there is no hope of him living for more than a few days, or that if he were to survive he would be so disabled that his quality of life would be unbearable, they will have discussions about whether it is in the baby's best interest to continue to give full intensive care.

If they reach the conclusion that continued intensive care is futile and likely to cause your baby unnecessary pain, the consultant will arrange a meeting to discuss their decision and the reasoning behind it with you. This is obviously a very difficult and distressing conversation, and it is important that you feel you have all the information you need and that you are not being rushed. Where possible, it is important for both parents to be at the meeting. Single mums will find the support of a close friend or family member invaluable.

Decision not to resuscitate Many neonatal units would say that 500g (1lb 2oz) is the limit of viability and so would not resuscitate a baby who weighed less than this. The limits for resuscitation vary across the UK and around the world, and these boundaries may be according to weight, length of gestation, or both. Some units outside the UK will not resuscitate babies who are born at less than 26 weeks, although many hospitals in the UK will resuscitate a baby born at 23 weeks if he's big enough. If a baby has been born extremely prematurely and doctors have to make a decision about whether or not to resuscitate him, weight is a helpful way to guide that decision.

If a baby is too small and premature to be considered viable, he may be wrapped up in a bundle and given to his mum and dad to hold. This may

---

TWINS AND TRIPLETS
When a twin is very ill

If you have twins or triplets who are born before 28 weeks, there is a higher risk than with single babies that at least one of them may have significant problems. In addition, with multiple births the delivery process is more complicated, so there is a greater chance of difficulties during birth.

After the birth, the contrast between a well twin and a sick one can be very hard for parents to cope with emotionally as well as practically. It

is particularly difficult when doctors have to sit down with parents and discuss the possibility that one of the twins may not survive. This is more likely to be the second twin.

When a baby dies on the unit, the family will be offered bereavement support. It's vital that when a twin has died, the family still receives this support, even though they have taken home a healthy baby. It's also important to remember that as the surviving twin grows up, he may be very curious about his sibling. Having photos and mementos to share with your child is a lovely way of remembering your baby together.

seem cruel, but resuscitating a 450g (1lb) baby will cause him pain and distress, and even if he gets through the first week, the chance of him surviving and having a good quality of life is very, very small.

Decisions about treatment
Staff on a neonatal unit – the doctors, the nurses, the chaplains, the psychotherapists, and others – work together as a team. Their regular meetings are sometimes used to talk about difficult decisions, such as whether it is appropriate to continue to give intensive care to a baby who has very severe brain damage and who is unlikely to have a reasonable quality of life in the future.

Making difficult decisions about treatment and explaining these to parents is one of the hardest things a paediatrician has to do. Doctors naturally want to protect parents from painful information, but it is vital that they are always honest. It's

The most important consideration in making an end-of-life plan is to avoid distress for the baby. Deciding on the correct pain relief would be a priority. For instance, morphine may be prescribed, because as well as giving excellent pain relief, it also gets rid of the discomfort the baby feels if he's in respiratory distress. A baby will always continue to be given expert nursing care and will be kept warm and comfortable.

When the plan is drawn up, everybody signs it and it will be distributed to anyone who needs to know about it. A plan like this is not a legal document – it simply expresses the wishes of the family and the professionals at that point in time and can be changed at any time, rather like a birth plan. Because these plans are made in partnership with parents, it's unusual for there to be major disagreements between families and the neonatal unit team.

> "I couldn't name him for two weeks. I thought, if I name him it becomes so real and what if something happens? If I don't, maybe I can get through."
>
> *Cher, mum to Xavier*

important that parents can trust the medical team to tell them the truth, even when it's very hard to hear. This is often emotionally draining for doctors as well as parents.

Sometimes there will be discussions around whether or not to continue ventilating a baby or, if a baby is no longer on a ventilator, should he be put back on if his condition deteriorates. These issues are all talked through very carefully and then the team will sit down with the baby's parents to discuss together what would be the most appropriate thing to do for the baby, depending on what happens. This is sometimes called an end-of-life plan, and essentially focuses on what care the baby will have.

What if parents and staff disagree?
The decision to withdraw intensive care is recommended to parents by the staff, but the team always works in partnership with parents. Therefore, if you disagree with this decision, the medical team will continue to give the baby full intensive care and will keep you fully updated of his progress so that the decision can be revisited if necessary.

Disagreements about withdrawing intensive care are entirely understandable. Some parents have religious reasons for not allowing withdrawal of care, while others don't want to give up hope in case a miracle happens. This rarely poses difficulties as the underlying principle of good care is to be honest with parents, and for the medical team to share their concerns and offer advice and guidance.

It is a parent's right to disagree. Very, very rarely, doctors will resort to going to court if they feel that the baby's quality of life is unbearable and his parents remain adamant that life should continue at all costs.

What happens next? If your consent isn't needed immediately, make sure you take your time in making your decision. It will give you the chance to think everything through and try to come to terms with what the doctors and nurses have told you.

If you agree with withdrawing intensive care, this does not mean that your baby will stop receiving

deep sadness are to be expected and may last for many months or years. The nurses and doctors on the unit will do their best to guide you through this very difficult time and to help you take the time you need to make decisions about what you would like to happen next.

Saying goodbye Spending time cuddling your baby in a quiet place away from intensive care is very important for many parents, and you should never feel that you are being hurried. You might like to bathe him and dress him or you may prefer the nurses to do that. The baby can stay with you overnight if you wish before being taken to the mortuary; if he goes to the mortuary you can come back to visit him later.

> " It's only now that I really say Alfie's name. Before I would say 'the baby'. I've got pictures, but it was like it happened to someone else. It never goes away. "
>
> *Claudia, mum to Chase*

excellent nursing care. It will mean, however, that your baby can be taken off the ventilator and given to you to cuddle. You may choose to stay with him in the unit or to spend time together in a quiet room.

He may continue to breathe for many hours or his heart may stop quickly after the ventilator is switched off. Whatever happens, this is a very precious time and should not be hurried.

When a baby dies There is nothing to compare with the relationship between a parent and child. Tragically, sometimes despite the best medical treatment, a baby is too premature or too sick to survive. When a baby dies, there is nothing that anyone can do or say to make things better for the parents. Feelings of anger, guilt, and

For some families it will be important to see the hospital chaplain or a religious leader of their faith, and this can be arranged by the nurses. For others, they may prefer to invite their own chaplain to visit and say prayers.

If your baby is not having a postmortem, you may like to ask the nurses in the unit if you can take him home before the funeral. This may be a time when you would like the extended family to visit and say goodbye to your baby. It's also an opportunity for the baby's siblings to cuddle him and understand he has died.

Keepsakes Many parents like to have photos taken of their baby, particularly if he has lived only for a very short time and they have not had a chance to take many photos themselves. It is also comforting to gather a collection of memories of your baby to be able to look at and touch in the years to come. These may include hand and foot prints, a lock of hair, the cot labels, blankets, the cuddly toy that was in the incubator with him, wristbands, and clothes he wore.

Why did my baby die?

Your consultant may ask you if you would like a postmortem to be carried out in order to find out more about the cause of death. Unless your baby died unexpectedly and the coroner has requested a postmortem, the decision about whether one is carried out will be yours to make. The procedure will be fully explained and you will be asked to sign a consent form to show that you have understood.

What about the funeral?

The hospital can arrange the funeral, and a burial or cremation, if that is what you would like, or you can arrange these yourselves. Sometimes undertakers will agree to provide a funeral for a baby free of charge.

Siblings may like to be involved with the planning of the funeral and may want to leave something special they have chosen with the baby. If they do want to do this, make sure it's not something they will miss later. If they come to the funeral it is helpful to arrange for a friend or relative to be there for them, so that they can take them out if it becomes too much for them.

Medical support for you

Your consultant will offer you a chance to meet up in a few days or weeks to check how you are, let you know the results of the postmortem if one was carried out, and answer any questions you may have.

If you were breastfeeding or expressing milk for your baby, your supply won't stop straight away. However, your doctor can prescribe some medicine that will make this happen more quickly.

MY STORY

Kamini says...

"I have had five pregnancies in total. The first and fourth I had early miscarriages. With my second pregnancy we lost our baby boy, Shaant, at 23 weeks. I went into premature labour after my waters breaking at 22 weeks. He only lived for one hour after I had delivered him.

The whole experience was very distressing. We only tried for another baby once I had medical tests to ensure that there wasn't an underlying reason why I couldn't carry a baby to term. The consultant gave me an action plan for my next pregnancy.

I fell pregnant for the third time quite soon after our loss. I continued to get counselling throughout the pregnancy as I found it hard to cope emotionally. I found it difficult to enjoy the pregnancy and felt a huge relief when my baby, Kamran, was born at term.

Having carried to term once I never expected our baby from my fifth pregnancy to be premature, but Jaden was born at 27 weeks, weighing 915g [2lb] . Deep down inside I never believed that he would make it until the day they said he was well enough to come home. In total, he spent 10 weeks on a neonatal unit.

We will never forget our baby Shaant that we lost, and I don't think that a day goes by that my husband and I do not think of him. After all we have been through, I am glad that we did not give up trying as we would never have had our two lovely boys Kamran and Jaden."

Kamini, mum to Jaden

Emotional support for you

In most areas, a bereavement counsellor will contact you, but your consultant will also be able to recommend where to seek emotional support, including counselling and local support groups.

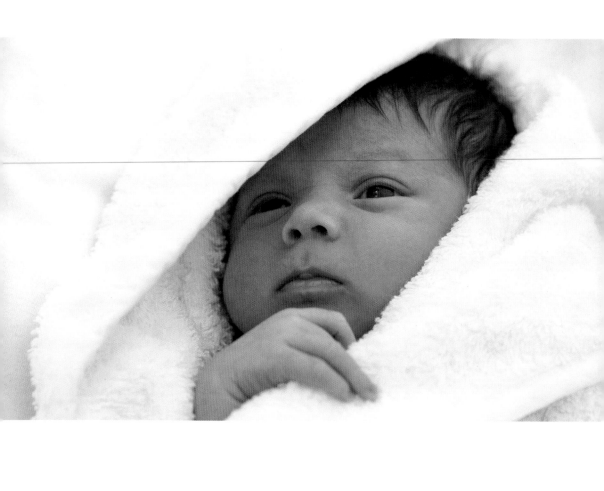

Going home

You've been longing to take your baby home, but when the time comes, you may feel apprehensive. Don't worry: the staff will make sure you and your baby are ready for the big day.

Preparing to take your baby home

The day you've been waiting for has finally arrived – your baby is well enough to leave hospital. You may be nervous as well as excited, but the staff will make sure you're ready to cope and that you know what support is available.

Preparing to take your baby home can be very exciting, and it's what you've been longing to do. It is also a big step, though, especially if she's been in the neonatal unit for a long time, and you might have mixed feelings about whether you're ready to cope. It is perfectly normal to feel apprehensive

baby can stay in the unit for a little longer to try to prepare themselves further. However, once your baby is ready to leave, then being at home with her parents is the best place for her to be.

Your baby will be ready to leave the unit when she's big enough to maintain her body temperature

> **"I was so excited to take him home but also terrified that the medical staff and equipment wouldn't be on hand."**
>
> *Kamini, mum to Jaden*

about caring for your baby at home, where the doctors and nurses and the technology won't be available around the clock. Parents often ask if their

TWINS AND TRIPLETS
Helping hands

Once you are home with twins or more, accept all offers of help. If friends ask what they can do to help, cooking, shopping, and making cups of coffee are all suggestions you can offer them!

With twins or more it's essential in the early weeks and months to be as organized as you possibly can and to have a rota of people who can come in and lend a hand.

If you don't have friends or family nearby, you could try asking your local nursery nursing college to see whether any of their final year students are looking for work experience placements.

in a normal environment, and usually when she's fully breastfed or bottle-fed, and will not need any special nursing care that you can't provide for her at home. Some babies go home tube fed with support.

If your baby is almost ready to be discharged, you may be worried about looking after her yourselves and not having anybody to ask about your concerns. The nurses will assess whether you're ready to take your baby home, so don't worry about not being able to cope – you won't be put in the position of taking her home until the staff feel confident that you will be able to care for her. If your baby will still need special care or certain medications once she's home, the nurses will ensure you are fully trained.

There is no set weight or age for discharge but most babies are at least 1.8kg (4lb), although they can be as small as 1.5kg (3lb 5oz). This is still very small, but as long as your baby is robust and well enough, then she will be fine to go home.

There will be quite a few things for you to prepare when your baby is ready to be discharged – both in

> "I've done rooming in for two nights. I slept an hour and a half the first night, and two hours the second!"
>
> *Sophie, mum to Samuel and Leo*

the last few days in the unit, and also at home (see the checklists on pp.88–89), and remember to ask the nurses if you are unsure of anything. You should also try to get as much rest as you can before the day of discharge, so you feel as relaxed and rested as possible.

Rooming in The thought of your baby leaving the security of the unit after many weeks or months can be overwhelming and frightening, especially if she still seems very small and vulnerable. In most units, you will be offered the chance to "room in",

which means spending a few nights in a room alone with your baby in order to have a chance to get used to doing everything yourselves, while still having the nurses on standby to answer any queries. This will include dressing her, changing her nappies, bathing her, and using any equipment that she still needs – like being at home, but with 24-hour support on hand if you need it. Rooming in will increase your confidence in caring for your baby by yourself, and will also give you an idea on what to expect once you are at home. Studies show that rooming in is a positive experience for parents.

Getting ready You may have mixed feelings on your baby's last day in the unit. Just remember that home is the best place for you all to be.

Warm and snug Make sure that your baby is wrapped up well for her journey home, as she will be used to the toasty temperature of the unit.

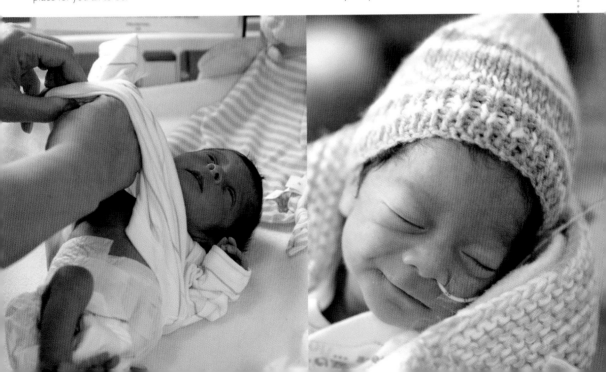

Checklists

Before you leave hospital, it's important for you to feel that you're ready to manage at home. If you're not sure about anything or you'd like to be shown again how to do something, ask the staff while your baby is still on the unit.

Before you leave the unit
Have you ...

✓ Changed your baby's nappy?

✓ Given your baby a bath?

✓ Learned how to store expressed breast milk?

✓ Learned how to make up formula feeds, if needed?

✓ Learned how to wash and sterilize bottles and teats?

✓ Been shown how to give your baby his medicine? If you don't feel confident, it's fine to ask again.

✓ Dressed your baby appropriately for the journey home?

✓ Arranged safe transport home for your baby?

✓ Been told about reducing the risk of cot death?

✓ Been shown basic first aid?

✓ Registered your baby with your GP? You will be given an NHS number for your baby while you're on the unit, and it's important to register him before you take him home.

✓ Registered the birth of your baby? This needs to be done within six weeks.

✓ Sorted out everything you'll need at home (see opposite)?

Baby clothes Make sure the clothes you buy for your baby are easy to put on and take off.

Car seat If you'll be travelling by car, you will need a first-stage car seat and a special insert for tiny babies.

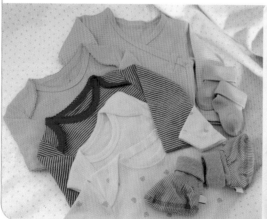
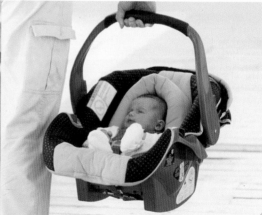

At home
What kit does my baby need?

Must haves:
- √ Nappies in the correct size.
- √ Clothes in your baby's size.
- √ Bottle-feeding and sterilizing equipment if your baby will have bottles.
- √ Cot and/or Moses baskets.
- √ Cot or pram-size sheets and blankets.
- √ Pram or buggy that lies flat and is suitable for a newborn.
- √ If you're going to be travelling by car, a first-stage infant car seat and a special insert to hold your tiny baby safely and securely.

If you like:
- √ Dummies – it's fine to use them and also fine not to.
- √ A small teddy or comforter, but don't put this in her cot as it can contribute to overheating.

Nappies If your baby is still tiny, extra small nappies are widely available to buy.

- √ Changing mat – or a towel will do.
- √ Baby bath – or a washing-up bowl will be fine.
- √ Changing bag – or use a small rucksack.

Check first:
- √ Gel pads and head rests – some babies have a tendency to hold their heads only to one side so that one side of the head becomes flat. Gel pads are available for these babies to lie on to help reshape their heads, but you should always ask your neonatal doctor or nurse whether these are advisable for your baby.

You don't need:
- ✕ Baby nests, warmers, wraps, and sheepskins, which can cause overheating.
- ✕ Sugar solution – this is given for pain relief on the unit, but your baby shouldn't have it at home as it can damage budding teeth.

Moses basket Make sure the mattress is the correct shape and size for your baby's basket or cot.

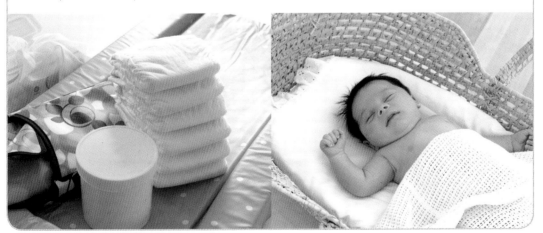

Going home on oxygen

Sometimes a baby is well enough to go home but may still need some extra oxygen. If your baby needs to go home on oxygen, you will be given all the kit, training, and support that you need.

The most common reason for a baby needing oxygen, even when she is well in other ways, is damage to the lungs caused by being on a ventilator or other form of respiratory support (see Chronic lung disease, p.78)

For how long will it be needed?

A baby who requires extra oxygen at home will need it until her lungs have healed. This may take a few months, but occasionally a baby will need the extra respiratory support for a few years. This might sound scary, but parents become used to the oxygen

Oxygen on the go If your baby needs extra oxygen, you will still be able to go out, and take the oxygen cylinders with you in a rucksack.

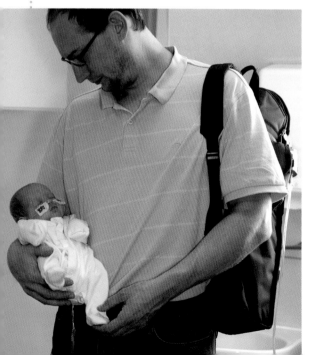

and the equipment very quickly, and it is rarely a problem. If your baby will need oxygen, the medical team will arrange for the necessary equipment to be installed. Don't be alarmed – it's normal to worry about giving oxygen initially, but you won't be asked unless the nurses feel that your baby is ready and are confident that you will be able to cope. There will also be community nurses to provide excellent support for you at home.

You will usually be given small oxygen cylinders that can go into a rucksack so you can get out and about with your baby. You can still go shopping or to the park, and visit family and friends if your baby is having oxygen.

How it works Oxygen at home can work in one of two ways. The oxygen normally comes from cylinders, with long tubes that connect to little nasal prongs that deliver the oxygen to your baby. The long tubes mean that you can move around with your baby. Cylinders are fine for babies who need oxygen intermittently for up to 12 hours a day. However, if your baby needs more oxygen than this, there is a device like a small, noisy fridge, which basically converts the air in the room into oxygen. This is called a concentrator, or compressor, and means that a continuous supply of oxygen is available and there is no need to keep replacing oxygen cylinders. As with cylinders, the oxygen is delivered to your baby by means of little prongs that fit into her nose. If your baby has a concentrator, you'll still be able to take her out and about with portable oxygen cylinders.

Setting it up If your baby goes home on oxygen, it will all be arranged for you, but exactly how it is organized will depend on how your individual neonatal unit works.

In some units, a company will be contacted to deliver the oxygen to your home and set it up so that it is ready for you to use. A nurse may go home with you and show you how to use the equipment and make sure that you understand how and when to administer the oxygen. She will also explain what to do if there is an emergency. Alternatively, the company who set up the equipment will come and show you how it works. Don't worry – whatever system your hospital has, somebody will be there to make sure you know what to do.

learn to look at her and see that she's okay, rather than relying on a machine. Parents generally get used to being without a monitor fairly quickly.

If your hospital can accommodate you, it may be worthwhile rooming in with your baby for a few nights before you go home, to practise getting used to being without a monitor.

Help and support If your baby is on oxygen at home, you'll have a particularly close relationship with the nurse who comes to see you. She will visit you regularly, and will adjust the concentration of oxygen your baby is receiving according to her needs. Whoever gives you support in the early weeks may see you until your baby is weaned onto

"Wherever he went, the oxygen went with him. There were tubes around the house, in the car... I didn't have a monitor, so I didn't know his sats levels – it was worrying."

Dana, mum to Erin and Max

Cautions The nurses will not only guide you on how to operate the oxygen machinery and how to give your baby the oxygen, but will also explain the potential hazards of having oxygen at home. Oxygen is a highly flammable gas, so you must make sure your baby and the oxygen equipment are kept well away from any open flames, such as a gas appliance with a pilot light. Radiators and heaters should be at least 1.5m (5ft) from the oxygen source. Parents (and visitors) must not smoke in the house.

Monitoring Normally when babies are ready to go home, they won't need an oxygen saturation monitor. It's normal for saturation levels to go up and down a lot, but changes can trigger the monitor's alarm to go off, which can cause anxiety. So when you're getting ready to take your baby home, and certainly once you are home, it's good to

air, although, depending on your area, the care of your baby may be transferred to a children's community team if this takes a very long time.

Weaning your baby onto air When the nurse or your community team thinks your baby is ready to be weaned off oxygen, they may bring a saturation monitor to your home so that the levels of oxygen in her blood can be recorded overnight. They will download this information onto a computer to see whether the oxygen your baby is having can be reduced or whether she is ready to stop using it altogether, and will discuss weaning your baby from oxygen onto air with you.

Weaning can be a slow process, occurring over several months, or it can happen within a matter of days, depending on how your baby responds and how confident you feel.

Sleep

Parents often worry about their baby's sleep. A routine will help him get used to the difference between night and day, and having his cot in the same room as you will mean you can keep a close eye on him.

Try to introduce the idea of day and night to your baby by changing him into nightclothes and keeping the room darker and quieter at night as this will slowly help him get used to the difference. Lots of babies don't like the dark and the silence at night as they are used to being on the ward and sleeping through things going on around them. So your baby may happily sleep all day while everyone's chatting and then at night he'll be wide awake.

Where should my baby sleep? Experts recommend that your baby sleeps in the same room as you for the first six months. He can sleep in a cot or a Moses basket next to your bed, although babies who are used to a small hospital cot may not like it if they're put into a big cot as soon as they get home. One option is to put a Moses basket inside the big cot until your baby is a bit older.

How warm should my baby be? Lots of parents are very concerned about room temperature when they're taking their babies home from hospital. This is partly because neonatal units are quite warm, especially the intensive care rooms, and so the recommended room temperature for a baby is lower than they are used to.

The Foundation for the Study of Infant Deaths (FSID) recommends that a baby's room should be between 16°C (61°F) and 20°C (68°F), so for a very small premature baby you might want to keep it towards the warmer end of this range. The general rule is to have the house temperature at whatever is comfortable for you, and then your baby will probably need one extra layer of clothing or blankets. If you're lying in bed sweltering with the heating on, then your baby is also too warm.

Overheating is just as much of a problem for premature babies as for term babies. Avoid making or buying nests like the ones on the unit as these will be too warm for your baby once he's at home. Some babies are so used to being wrapped that they will settle better if they're swaddled, and if this is the case with your baby you can wrap him with a single sheet – don't use a blanket. When your baby is older, a baby sleeping bag can be useful as you can zip him in and he can't lose his bedding. It's important that you buy one that's the right size for

Back to sleep Always put your baby on his back to sleep, and make sure his feet are at the foot of his cot so he can't wriggle under the covers and overheat.

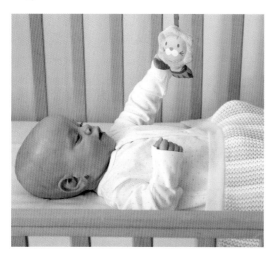

your baby's weight though, so that he can't slip down inside it and overheat.

Breathing monitor All new parents worry when they take their tiny baby home for the first time, and if he's spent time in special care it can feel even more scary. You might be frightened that he'll stop breathing (apnoea), or feel panicky about cot death and infections.

Babies thought by staff to be at significant risk of apnoea may be offered a monitor. However, this is rare as the medical staff will not send your baby home until they feel that it is safe to do so. Doctors don't recommend apnoea monitors in general, but some parents buy one nevertheless. Usually they don't use them for very long.

There are steps that all parents can take to reduce the risk of cot death (see below). Depending on your baby's medical problems, there may be an increased

risk of cot death, and this is something the medical team on the neonatal unit will discuss with you. You may be offered a scheme known as CONI-plus. CONI stands for "care of next infant" and is normally offered to parents who have lost a baby to cot death. CONI-plus is for parents whose baby is at increased risk due to medical concerns.

Noisy breathing It is normal for premature babies to breathe very noisily. The typical premature baby sound is a sort of snuffly, squeaky sound and it can worry parents a lot, especially in the middle of the night. As a parent of a premature baby on the unit, you may not notice these sounds when there are monitors beeping and people talking around you, but they can seem extremely loud in a quiet room. If you are worried or your baby appears to be having difficulty breathing, ask a health professional for advice.

NEED TO KNOW

Reducing risk of cot death

Cot death, also called sudden infant death syndrome (SIDS), is a worry for all new parents, but the following measures help reduce the risk:

● Place your baby's cot next to your bed: don't have your baby in bed with you. The risks of sharing a bed with their parents are increased for premature or small-for-dates babies.

● Put your baby on his back to sleep at night and during naps.

● Make sure your baby's feet are at the foot of the cot so he can't wriggle down and get his head under the bedclothes, which can cause him to overheat.

● Use a firm mattress and avoid using a duvet, pillows, and toys in the cot.

● Don't let your baby get too warm. It's fine if your baby's hands or feet are cool, but if his tummy or neck is hot or sweaty, remove a layer or two of his bedding. Always take off his hat and extra clothing when you come indoors.

● If you are tempted to bring your baby into your bed when he is older, don't do this if you or your partner smoke, or if you have been drinking, have taken medication that could make you drowsy, or if you're very tired.

● Don't fall asleep on the sofa or in an armchair with your baby.

● Particularly with a premature baby, always take him out of the car seat when you're not in the car.

● Keep your baby away from smoky places and ensure nobody smokes in your home.

● If your baby is unwell, seek medical advice straight away.

Feeding your baby at home

Whether your baby is having your milk from the breast or bottle, or having infant formula, she will be getting all the nutrients she needs to grow stronger, and milk will be the most important part of her diet for the first year.

In most cases, babies go home with breastfeeding and/or bottle-feeding already established. However, some babies will have a nasogastric tube still in place, and you'll be shown how to manage this before your baby leaves the unit.

You don't have to feed your baby upright or wind her in certain positions unless the medical team has given you specific instructions.

How often? Babies can become quite institutionalized and tend to be in a routine in the unit. This can be helpful as it means that when your baby comes home she is likely to be feeding three- or four-hourly and sleeping regularly. However, this is not always the case and it's entirely normal for babies to abandon their routine and have random feeding and sleeping patterns.

Once she comes home, you can just feed her on demand – she'll let you know when she's hungry. If she was very premature, she'll be more regimented than if she was just a little bit early and hasn't been on the unit for so long. If she was only on the unit for a short period of time, she'll probably be demand feeding quite quickly.

How much? On average, a newborn baby, once established on feeds, is going to need around 150ml per kg (5oz per lb) of body weight per day. This is impossible to measure if you're breastfeeding, but if you're bottle-feeding, it's a good idea to add up at the end of each day how much you've given your baby. If you're giving her 200ml per kg (7oz per lb) per day and she's vomiting all the time, it's probably because you're giving her too much! If you're giving her 120ml per kg (4oz per kg) per day and she's vomiting all the time and not growing, talk to your neonatal nurse, health visitor, or GP.

Milk contains all the fluid your baby needs, so there is usually no need to give her extra water or juice. You can tell that your baby is doing well if she's gaining weight at a reasonable rate, sucking for a good amount of time, has several wet nappies each day, is alert, and looks well.

TWINS AND TRIPLETS
Feeding more than one

If your twins or triplets are established at the breast, it may be possible for you to breastfeed two babies simultaneously, saving a lot of time. Or you could breastfeed one baby and bottle-feed the others with expressed breast milk or formula, then alternate for the next feed.

If your babies are on the same feeding and sleeping schedule, this will hopefully make life a bit easier for you, especially if you feed one baby and your partner the other. It's perfectly normal for multiples to feed and sleep at different times, though, so enlist as much help as you can, and be prepared by expressing and storing breast milk when possible.

Time for two If you want to breastfeed your twins at the same time, try tucking a baby under each arm. Special cushions are available to get them into the right position.

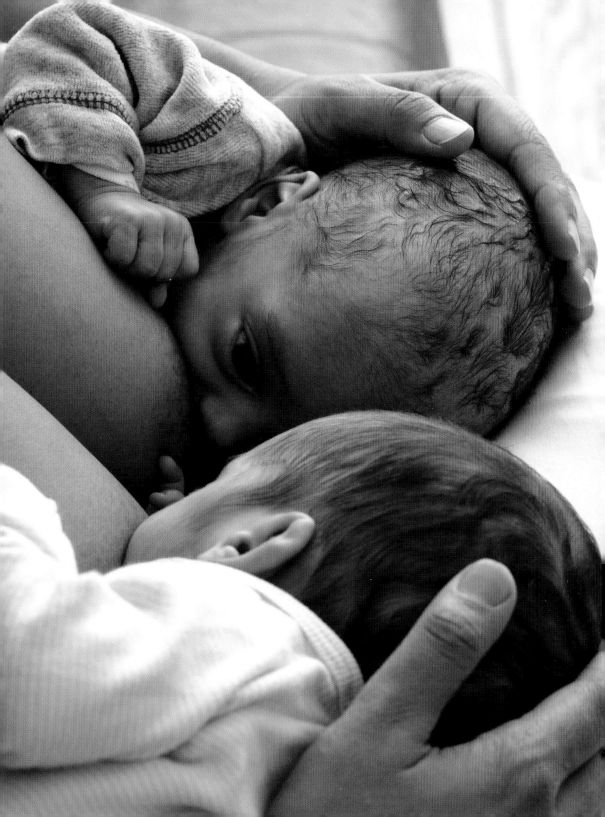

Which milk should my baby have?

Mums are encouraged to breastfeed where possible and most babies will go home fully breastfed. A few babies will be given some form of pre-term formula if this has been advised by a dietician in order to help with weight gain or if you have been unable to produce enough milk to fully breastfeed your baby. Pre-term formula aims to provide your baby with nutrients similar to those found in breast milk.

everyone. If you haven't been able to express and/or breastfeed, or if your baby was born very early and you've been expressing for months and want to stop, your baby will still receive the necessary nutrition.

When your baby reaches around a month or so after she was due to be born, she may be able to switch to an ordinary newborn formula. Depending on the system where you live, this may be a

> " Chase had the worst reflux I've ever seen – projectile vomiting every time I fed him. It improved when he went onto solids. "
>
> *Claudia, mum to Chase*

If you're expressing breast milk for tube feeds, and there isn't enough of your milk, breast milk from a donor breast-milk bank or formula is given instead. Lots of mums with premature babies express and then successfully breastfeed, but it's not easy for

discussion you have with your community nurse, your health visitor, or a dietician. They will look at your baby's growth and weight gain with you, and the decision will be based on this and any other health issues your baby has.

When you make up bottles of formula, it's important that you follow the instructions on the pack exactly – always add the correct amount of milk powder to the bottle. Pre-term formula in hospital is often ready mixed, but you will be shown how to make up a bottle with powdered formula while you're on the unit.

If your baby has only ever had breast milk, you may find that she doesn't tolerate formula very well, especially the pre-term formula, which is not so easy to digest. This can sometimes lead to problems with reflux, in which the stomach contents come back up into the oesophagus (gullet), or with constipation. Sometimes when you think your baby is constipated, there isn't a problem after all. It's just that different milks produce poos of different consistency. However, if, for any reason, you think your baby isn't tolerating her formula, discuss this with your health visitor or GP.

TIPS
Coping with reflux

- Try to keep your baby upright when feeding.
- Prop her cot up by putting something under the legs at the head of the cot. Or you could try placing a rolled-up blanket or towel under the mattress, but make sure this is actually propping up your baby rather than ending up as a pillow.
- Offer smaller but more frequent feeds.
- Reflux medicine is supposed to be given just before a feed. Have the medicine ready before you need it and give it to your baby as soon as she wakes up. Then when it's time to feed her, you'll be ready to give her milk straight away rather than trying to get medicine down a frantically hungry, crying baby.

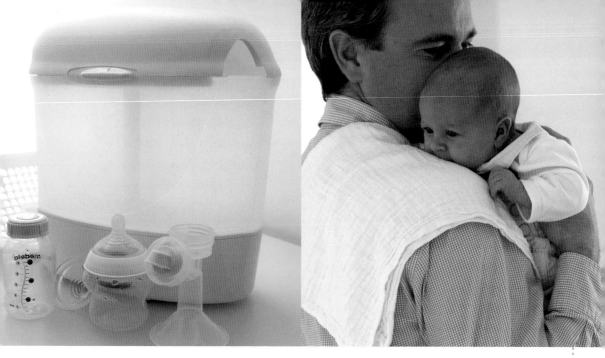

Sterilizing Sterilize your baby's feeding equipment for the first few months to limit the risk of infection. Make sure you wash off all traces of milk first.

Help for reflux If your baby suffers from reflux, simple strategies such as holding her upright, can help. Only babies with severe symptoms need medication.

Which bottles should I use? Get whatever bottles suit your baby best – any type is fine – but you'll need to buy special, soft teats that are recommended for premature babies.

By the time your child has finished with bottles, you'll probably have been through every make of bottle and teat because what suits her one month won't necessarily suit her next month. Don't worry that you've wasted money on buying them as at some stage they'll probably be just right for her!

It's important to wash a baby's bottles and teats thoroughly in hot, soapy water and rinse them well. Use a bottle brush to get every bit of milk out. When your baby comes home from hospital, you'll also need to sterilize her feeding equipment as she's vulnerable to infection. You can use an electric steam sterilizer, a microwave sterilizer, or cold-water chemicals to do this. Or you can boil the items in a pan for at least 10 minutes, making sure that everything stays under the water. If using chemicals, don't rinse the bottles and teats when you take them out as this will mean they are no longer sterile.

Reflux Gastro-oesophageal reflux, in which the immature valve at the top of your baby's stomach does not close properly and allows milk to come back up, is very common in premature babies. The regurgitated milk contains stomach acids, which can make your baby's oesophagus (gullet) very sore.

The severity of reflux differs for every baby, but common symptoms include excessive vomiting, crying after feeding, and acute coughing. If your baby has reflux, she may dislike lying flat, especially after feeds. In the unit, the cot bases can be tilted to prop her up, but when you get home you can improvise (see box, left). Reflux can be miserable for your baby and for you, but try not to worry. It can be treated and she will eventually grow out of it.

Medication

When your baby was in the unit, the nurses would have administered any necessary medication. Now your baby is at home, you are responsible for ensuring he receives the correct dosage and at the right time.

Before you leave the hospital, someone will go through all your baby's medicines with you to make sure you know exactly what each one is for and how and when to give it to him. If there's anything you don't understand, ask.

Babies often leave hospital with lots of different types of medicine, which may need to be given at different times of the day.

Types of medicine Lots of premature babies suffer from reflux and many babies will be sent home from the unit on anti-reflux medication. These medicines can include antacids, thickeners, drugs that help reduce acid production in the stomach, and drugs that increase the rate at which milk leaves the stomach so there is less milk left to come up again. Reflux medicines may have to be

> " I struggled in the first few days to get all the timings right. I drew a chart, which helped me keep on track. "
>
> *Kamini, mum to Jaden*

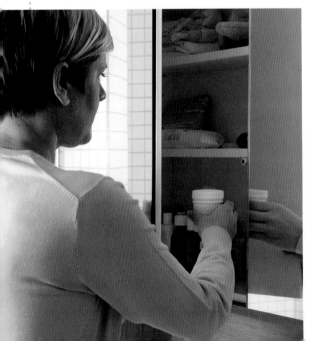

Taking charge Try to stay as organized as possible if your baby requires medication. Keep the bottles in the same place and note how much medicine remains.

given three or four times a day. For more about reflux and tips on coping with this see pages 96–97.

A few babies are sent home on diuretics, which help the kidneys to get rid of any excess fluid in the body. These may be given to babies who have chronic lung disease or a heart problem.

Sometimes your baby will be prescribed eye or nose drops.

Giving your baby medicine It's not always easy to administer medicine to a small baby, so it helps to have an action plan before you start!
Oral medication Your baby's medication is likely to be in a liquid form, which you give with a special oral medicine syringe. Here's how to do it:
● Draw the medicine up into the syringe until you have the required number of millilitres (if you have this prepared before your baby needs it, you're less likely to feel flustered when it's time to give it).

- Hold your baby securely and comfortably as this will help him (and you) stay calm and relaxed.
- Put the tip of the syringe into the corner of his mouth and encourage him to suck it as you gently squirt the medicine in.
- Aim for the inside of his cheek, not the back of his throat, so that he doesn't gag.
- If your baby is finding this difficult, try putting a bottle teat into his mouth and squirting the medicine into that as he may find it easier to suck it through the teat.
- If you're having any problems giving your baby his medicine, talk to your community nurse or health visitor. If you are concerned that your premature baby is unwell, seek medical help rather than giving him over-the-counter medicines.

Eye or nose drops These can be especially tricky to administer, and it's always easier to do it if you have someone to help you. To give eye drops, wrap your baby in a towel to prevent flailing arms and lay him in your lap. Hold his head steady and pull his lower lid down slightly. Place one drop into each eye

TIPS
Keeping track

- Make a chart, with little squares for each dose of each medicine your baby has during the day. Tick off each one as you give it.
- Try to have the medicine ready to give your baby in advance so you're not trying to get everything ready when your baby is crying for a feed.
- Avoid giving your baby medication at night wherever possible. For instance, reflux medication will generally be three to four times a day, so if you give the first dose after 6am and the last dose before 10pm you shouldn't need to be giving anything in the middle of the night. This will help your baby get used to there being very little going on at night.

formula, he may not need supplements as this usually contains all the vitamin and iron supplements a premature baby needs. Many babies are discharged from the unit on special

> "The medicine side was quite scary because I had a lot of syringes to give, and in hospital the nurses had always done it. Now I had to give all this medication."
> *Dana, mum to Erin and Max*

behind the lower lid. Repeat if he blinks and you don't think the drop went in.

To give nose drops, hold your baby as you would to give eye drops, tilt his head back, and place a drop in each nostril.

Vitamins and minerals If your baby was born at less than 35 weeks he'll be given vitamins, iron, and folic acid supplements, and if you're breastfeeding he'll have these even if he was born after 35 weeks. If your baby is having a pre-term

post-discharge formula milk that contains more vitamins and minerals than normal infant formula. It's a good idea to check with your GP or health visitor which iron or vitamin supplements he will need once he switches to ordinary infant formula.

Current UK guidelines recommend that all children have vitamin supplements containing vitamins A and D until the age of five.

Some very premature babies are also sent home with phosphate supplements. These are given to promote healthy bone development.

Everyday care

The practical care you give your baby at home will be the same as in the unit, so you will have had plenty of practice. You'll soon discover which nappies work best for you and your baby and ways to make bath time enjoyable.

Generally, if your baby is well enough to go home she will be robust enough to be looked after in the same way that is advised for babies born at term. The only exception is if the medical team has given you specific instructions about certain aspects of her care – if she is on oxygen or still has a nasogastric tube, for instance.

You will have learned to bath her, dress her and change nappies while she was in hospital, so practical care won't be as much of a challenge as it is for parents of term babies who bring them home straight away after the birth.

Caring for two When caring for twins on your own, change and bath one baby at a time, while keeping the other one nearby.

Nappies You can now use baby wipes instead of cooled, boiled water for changing your baby's nappy, although cooled, boiled water is fine. Use whichever nappies suit you and your baby best.

There are several brands of disposable nappies that come in sizes small enough for premature babies, and these are widely available in many chemists and supermarkets.

If you prefer reusables, you can find shaped cloth nappies for babies from around 2.5kg (5lb) in weight. Some makes have a separate nappy and an outer wrap, while others are all in one. You can also use traditional terry nappies but you'll need to fold them so they're small enough to fit on a tiny baby. Whichever type you use, a disposable liner inside will help to protect your baby's bottom.

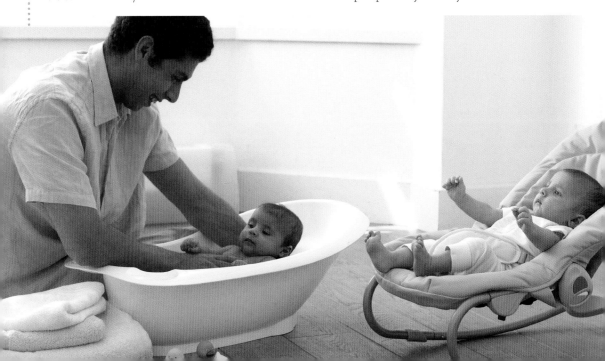

Keeping your baby clean Your baby doesn't need frequent baths, and topping and tailing (washing her face, hands, and nappy area) will be fine on the days you don't bath her. It's still a good idea to use a new piece of gauze or cotton wool (this is fine to use now) with cooled, boiled water to wash each eye for the first few weeks. You don't need to use soap or bath liquid to wash the rest of her, but if you do, ensure they are specially formulated baby products as other toiletries can irritate her skin.

Baby massage Parents have been massaging their babies for centuries. It's a lovely way to feel close to and communicate with your baby. It can also help her to sleep better.

Choose a time when your baby is calm and relaxed and make sure that the room is warm so she won't feel chilly. Lay her on a soft surface on her back with a nappy or towel under her. If she's uncomfortable being naked, leave her clothes on. You don't need oil, but if you do use it, avoid aromatherapy and nut oils. Organic sunflower oil is a good option.

A few minutes are long enough at first. Try massaging her arms and legs, from shoulders to hands and thighs to feet, or her tummy, by rubbing her abdomen lightly in a clockwise direction, working outwards from her belly button. Use light, circular strokes on her head, avoiding the fontanelles, then stroke the sides of her face. On her chest, gently stroke from top to bottom. When you have massaged her front, turn her onto her tummy and massage her back, stroking from her head downwards.

If your baby seems unhappy, stop. She'll let you know if she's had enough by turning her head away, shutting her eyes tightly, whimpering, or crying. Ask your health visitor or community nurse for more information about massage techniques or classes if you're unsure.

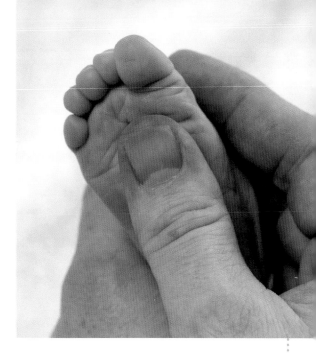

Soothing touch Lots of babies love being massaged. Both you and your baby may find it relaxing and an enjoyable way to bond.

How often should your baby poo?

Parents often worry about this when they take their babies home. The important thing to remember is that your baby doesn't need to poo every day, and some babies, especially if they're breastfed, may go for a few days without doing a poo. As long as your baby is feeding and seems well, you don't need to worry. If the colour of her poo changes (see p.67), then have it checked by your doctor.

If you are moving on from breast milk to formula, your baby might become constipated at first as the formula is harder for her to digest. Try giving her a little cooled, boiled water, just as you would with a term baby. It's important that you don't give her more than 10–15ml (3–4tsp), though, because otherwise you'll fill her tummy up and she won't drink as much milk as she needs. If you think your baby may be constipated, talk to your community nurse, health visitor, or GP.

You and your baby

Spending time with your baby is brilliant for both of you. You are your baby's whole world and the bond between you will keep growing. As his personality unfolds, your time together will become more and more rewarding.

Playing and interacting with your baby is one of the lovely aspects of early parenthood and is very enjoyable for both of you, so don't miss out. There are lots of groups you can go along to, including get-togethers with other parents of babies who have had neonatal care. Your hospital or health visitor should have details of these.

It's fine to take your baby out and about – if he's well enough to be home, he's well enough to go out in a sling (if he's big enough) or in the pram or car. Bear in mind that all new babies need to lie flat, so it's important that you choose a pram or buggy that is suitable for a newborn. He'll need to be kept warm, so make sure he's wrapped up snugly when you go out and remember to put a hat on him as a lot of heat is lost through the head.

Will I struggle to bond? When your baby has been under the care of the medical team in hospital since his birth, you may find it strange when you finally get him home and are solely responsible for looking after him. This is not uncommon – you've been through such a traumatic time and have been entirely dependent on the nurses for your baby's care, often for many weeks.

It may have been very difficult bonding with your baby through the Perspex wall of the incubator in the neonatal unit. If you were scared your baby might die, you may have held back for fear of losing

Dad time Sometimes dads feel left out in the early days. Your baby will love having your full attention and your relationship will grow as you spend quality time together.

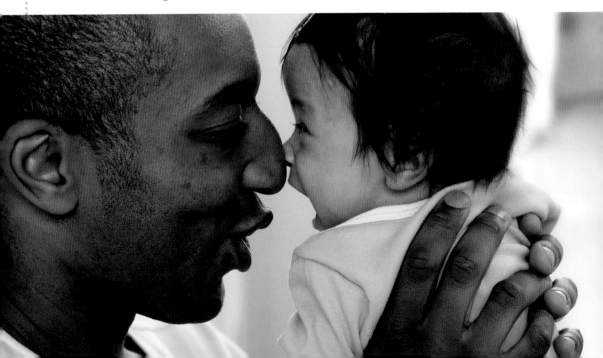

him. This is completely normal and hopefully the nurses will have encouraged you to get involved as much as possible while he was in the unit. However, it is understandable to feel anxious about your relationship with your baby and nervous of handling him and of the responsibility that being a parent entails. Rest assured that your baby will already have bonded with you through your touch, voice, and smell, and you will always be the best people to care for him and love him.

Enjoying your baby

Even a very tiny baby will enjoy time with you and playing gentle games, such as peek-a-boo. Even if he doesn't appreciate the games yet, he'll enjoy the interaction. Babies are fascinated by faces, especially yours, so hold him facing you and chat or sing to him. He'll also love it if you mimic his expressions and he may try to mimic yours, too!

When your baby cries

Premature babies don't cry very much, but now your baby is older he will start to use crying to communicate with you. His ways of telling you what he wants are very limited, so he'll cry if he is hungry, tired, uncomfortable, bored, or in need of a cuddle. As you get to know him better, you will recognize the difference between his cries and be able to respond quickly and, as a result, he will gradually cry less. There are plenty of ways to comfort your crying baby. Try the following:
- Motion – put him in the sling and walk around with him; or go out in the car as long as you are not too stressed to drive safely.
- White noise – place him in front of the washing machine on a spin cycle or next to a de-tuned radio.
- Try a dummy if he needs to suck.
If your baby is crying a lot and you're worried, or you feel you're not coping, seek advice from your community health team.

Advice from others

While your baby was in hospital and being looked after by medical staff, you friends and relatives probably did not feel they could interfere. But now that your baby is at home, you may find that you are suddenly inundated with doting grandparents, friends, and various random strangers, giving their views on what is best for your baby. Although well-meant and sometimes useful, a lot of this advice will be conflicting and leave you wondering exactly how to proceed.

While it is worth being tactful with grandparents, even if you don't agree with their views on childcare, it is important to start believing in yourselves as parents and doing things your way. You may make mistakes, but as you get to know your baby and how he responds to things, you will find out for yourselves the best way to care for him. Sources of advice on all aspects of life with a new baby include parenting books, magazines, and websites. You can also chat to your health visitor or GP.

TIPS

Paperwork

- Registering your baby's birth – you need to do this within six weeks even if your baby is still in hospital. If you have missed the six-week deadline, phone your local registry office and ask what you should do. You won't get child benefit until you have registered your baby.
- Your baby's NHS number – you will be given this, along with your baby's "Red Book", which is his personal child health record, while you are still in the unit.
- Registering with your GP – your baby won't automatically be registered with the GP because you are; you'll need to take his "Red Book" and NHS number to the GP's surgery and register him.

Friends and family

Once your baby is home, it's lovely to have visitors, but you may worry that she'll be exposed to infection. There are simple steps you can take to minimize this, and remember that trusted visitors could make good babysitters!

People will want to visit you and your baby at home, which is great if you feel up to it. It's natural to be concerned about your baby catching all the viruses that do the rounds. It's sensible to avoid mixing with people who have viral infections, if possible, as she will be more vulnerable to these than a healthy, term baby. For instance, a nasty cold can easily turn into bronchiolitis (see p.107) in a tiny baby, so don't worry about asking a cold-ridden friend or relative to delay their visit.

Time for you For any new parents, taking time out for yourselves is very important. When you've been through the turmoil of having a premature or sick baby, this can seem impossible, but if you can manage it, you and your baby will benefit.

It can be very hard to trust someone to look after your vulnerable baby, especially when she is still very tiny and you're just getting used to caring for her yourself. In addition, other people may be frightened to babysit if your baby still seems fragile.

> " I didn't take him to crowded places in the beginning, but ultimately you have to, and they can get colds anywhere. You just have to be sensible really. "
>
> *Claudia, mum to Chase*

While it's impossible to avoid your baby having contact with family members, if you have an older child who is unwell, it's best for him not to kiss or cuddle the baby until he's better. Toys shared with an older sibling who has a cold should be washed.

Good handwashing for everyone is important, especially if anyone has a cold.

Also, it is very important to keep premature babies away from cigarette smoke. Nobody should smoke in the house and, if possible, family members should try not to smoke at all, because the particles cling to your clothes, hair, and breath. Giving up smoking also reduces the risk of cot death (sudden infant death syndrome) as well as all sorts of respiratory issues. There's a very close association between wheezy children and smoking parents.

If you do have a family member or friend who can care for her for a short time, take the opportunity, even if it's just to go to a local café.

If you really can't find a way to go out alone or as a couple, for example in the early days of your baby being on oxygen, try to take the odd hour off to have a long, luxurious bath and read your book while your partner or a friend looks after the baby. If you're feeling down, anxious, and struggling with day-to-day life, talk to your community neonatal nurse, health visitor, or GP, as postnatal depression can occur several months after birth.

Lowering the risk When you have visitors, remind them that your baby is still vulnerable and stress the need for clean hands, even for your youngest guests.

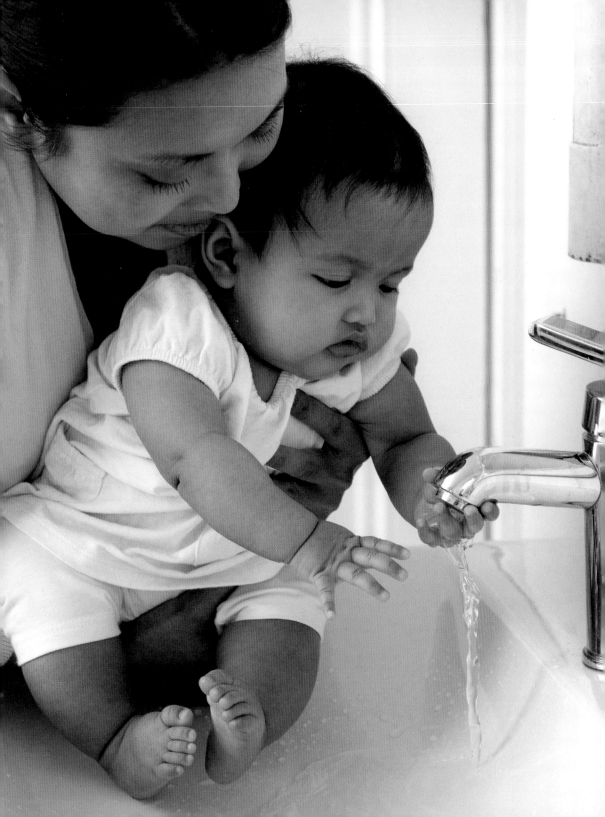

When you're worried

Your baby will have regular check-ups and visits from health professionals, but this won't stop you worrying that he might become ill. There are certain signs to watch out for, but if you're ever unsure then ring your doctor.

If your baby is considered to be particularly vulnerable, a nurse will visit regularly when you're at home, and you will be provided with a list of phone numbers to ring if you have any concerns. Your GP will be told that you're bringing your baby home (make sure you've registered the baby with your GP) and the health visitor will be in touch as well. So although you might feel quite isolated and worried to begin with, there are people on hand to help.

your baby's progress as he grows. They can offer advice about caring for your baby, immunizations, health and developmental worries, and any other concerns you might have.

Your health visitor will be able to give you details of local baby groups, postnatal support groups, baby

> " I'd seen such dreadful things: he nearly died so many times, so a snotty nose didn't seem like much. You worry about what you need to – I knew when things were serious. "
>
> *Claudia, mum to Chase*

clinics, and how to get to know other parents of special care babies. There are charities that run a network of support groups for families of premature and sick babies across the UK (see p.124).

Support for you Different areas offer different kinds of support for you and your baby when you take him home from hospital. In most places, babies under 34 weeks or weighing less than 2kg (4lb 3oz) when they are discharged will come under the care of either the neonatal community service, who will see you on the neonatal unit and at home, or the children's community nursing service. Babies who are older and bigger than this but who are on oxygen or who need any other care will also be seen by a nurse from one of these services.

Your health visitor will also make contact with you and come to visit once your baby is home. Health visitors are nurses who have had additional training in child health and development and will monitor

When to call the doctor If any baby has a fever – a raised temperature – in the first few months of life, you should always call for medical help because you don't know if it may develop into something to worry about.

With a young baby don't just guess: take his temperature to check whether it's raised. You can use forehead strips, which are simple to use and inexpensive. However, ear thermometers are more accurate and also quick and easy to use; they come with a disposable tip. They're a little more expensive than forehead strips but are a good investment. You should also call for medical help if your baby has any of the following symptoms:

- Excessive irritability much of the time

- Sweating a lot when feeding
- Not feeding properly – taking less than half his normal formula feeds or stopping more quickly than usual if you're breastfeeding
- Vomiting large amounts
- Not having as many wet nappies as usual
- Drowsiness, floppiness, lethargy, or not waking for feeds.

You should seek urgent medical help if your baby has any of the following:
- Colour change – blue, purple, or pale
- Fast breathing
- Difficulty breathing or wheezing
- Apnoea (stopping breathing)
- Unresponsiveness.

Trust your instincts. If you are worried that something isn't right, even if you can't quite put your finger on what's worrying you, see a doctor or speak to the community health team straight away. If you need to, call an ambulance.

Bronchiolitis Premature babies are at increased risk of getting an illness called bronchiolitis, which causes inflammation of the bronchioles, the smallest airways in the lungs. The illness is dominant in the autumn and winter, and babies on oxygen are particularly vulnerable.

Bronchiolitis is usually caused by a virus called RSV (respiratory syncytial virus). The viruses that cause bronchiolitis can affect anyone at any stage of life. However, in older children and adults these viruses will just give them a cold, whereas babies who are infected may develop bronchiolitis. Symptoms include:
- Wheezing
- A distinctive rasping cough
- A raised temperature
- Going off feeds – this happens because the baby is not be able to suck properly at the same time as breathing.

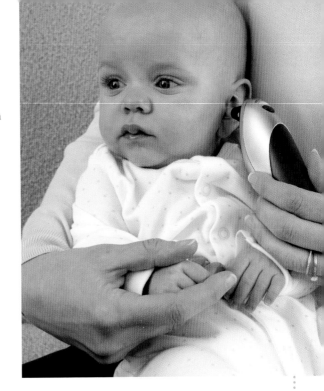

Temperature check Take your baby's temperature to find out whether he has a fever. An ear thermometer is easy to use, accurate, and quick.

If your baby develops any or all of these symptoms, take him to a doctor. If his lips turn blue or purple or he is struggling to breathe, call an ambulance.

There is no specific treatment, but a significant number of babies who have bronchiolitis need to be admitted to hospital for oxygen and help with feeds.

Meningitis This infection of the membranes that cover the brain can be caused by viruses or bacteria. Bacterial meningitis can cause long-term problems if it's not treated promptly. Symptoms in a baby can include a high-pitched or weak cry; bulging fontanelle; vomiting; irritability, drowsiness and floppiness; a rash or blotchy, clammy skin. The characteristic rash of dark spots that don't fade when pressed with a glass may not appear. If you suspect meningitis, seek medical help urgently.

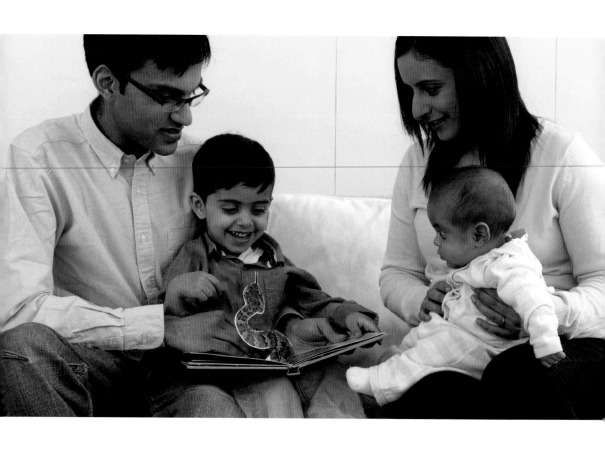

What the future holds

You and your baby have been through a lot and your bond is strong. He may have some catching up to do, but you can help him reach his full potential.

What follow-up will my baby have?

After your baby leaves the neonatal unit, she'll have regular health checks and she may also require more specialist follow-up care, depending on her medical and developmental needs.

The doctors will decide whether or not your baby needs any follow-up after leaving hospital. Your health visitor will come to see you and your baby whether you are having follow-up or not, and you will be invited to the baby clinic for check-ups with your GP. Depending on her gestation, development, and medical needs, your baby may also be visited at home by a community nurse, who will monitor her growth and any symptoms of concern (see p.106).

For some babies born after 31 weeks or so and with no medical concerns when they leave the unit, no specialist hospital or community follow-up is necessary. Although it may seem scary to go home and not be offered a hospital appointment, it signifies that the medical team do not think that long-term problems are likely and want you to treat your baby like any other healthy infant.

Six-week check All babies who are born at term and go straight home will have a six-week check-up with their GP, who will look at and ask about various aspects of their development.

When babies have been born prematurely, some GPs will do the check when babies are actually six weeks old if they're home, even if they were born early. Others will wait until around their corrected gestational age – so six weeks after their due date.

Hospital follow-up If necessary, your baby will be offered an appointment with the consultant at the hospital. If she spent the first part of her care at a level three neonatal unit (see p. 28) and then

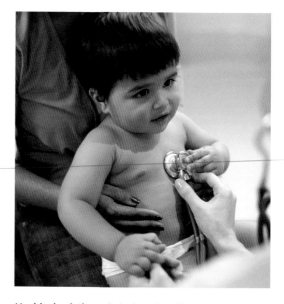

Health check If your baby has a lot of health checks after leaving hospital, he'll get used to being examined by the doctor and may be quite relaxed when being checked.

moved to a hospital nearer home, she might be offered follow-up appointments at both centres. If she had surgery, she may also be offered follow-up at the hospital where that was done.

Some babies may simply need to return to the hospital for one clinic appointment so that the medical team can do some blood tests and advise on whether certain treatments and medications need to be continued. If your baby was born very prematurely she will usually also be offered a hospital appointment to check her development when she's a year old.

Some babies require specialist follow-up, with the length of follow-up depending on the particular problem or problems; for example, all the smallest and sickest babies will be followed up by an ophthalmologist owing to the risk of retinopathy of prematurity (ROP) (see p.72). Some babies with complex issues, such as severe brain injury or heart problems that need surgery, may require life-long specialist follow-up.

Coordinating your baby's care If your baby has a number of specialists managing her medical care it can be overwhelming, and often parents feel as if they are the only ones coordinating everything. Ideally you should have one clinician whose role it is to take this responsibility. This may be your GP, paediatrician, or a specialist nurse. It usually doesn't matter who it is as long as he or she is someone with access to all the relevant information and to the other professionals looking after your baby. He or she also needs to be easily accessible to you when you have a query.

What's my baby's outlook? As soon as you discover your baby has a problem and she is admitted to the neonatal unit, you will be worrying about what the future holds. Parents often ask if their child will have any developmental difficulties, for example in walking or talking, and how long they will have to wait to find out. The answers to such questions will vary hugely, and subtle difficulties may take a long time to develop.

Ultrasound scanning and, in some cases, MRI scans of the brain can provide doctors with a great deal of useful information about the kind of problems your baby may encounter in the future. If major problems are anticipated you will be informed and updated. The only way of knowing for certain, however, about your baby's long-term development is to wait and see.

MY STORY
Claudia says...

"Chase still has ophthalmology, audiology, every 'ology'. I remember the consultant saying to me, 'Don't expect him to be totally unscathed by all this – there will be repercussions of his early birth.' At the time, I didn't see it – he was a perfect-looking baby, he didn't look ill at all.

He developed relatively normally physically. He was sitting, walking – he tippy-toe walked (and still does) – but physically everything looked fine. He had laser eye surgery when he was still in the hospital. He should wear glasses, but he just eats them so he is short-sighted, nothing severe.

But when I expected him to start babbling at around a year, there was just nothing. He started to play with things in an unusual way. If you've been around children, you know how they play: they take a car and roll it across the floor. They don't just look at the wheels going round and round and round. It was very repetitive, very unusual behaviour. He was also showing signs of lack of communication and imaginary play.

He was given a diagnosis of severe autism and global developmental delay. It's a very unclear line, and his is not a typical, classic case of autism. I think his problems are more on the developmental delay side than the autistic side, but he definitely has autistic traits. He's totally non-verbal.

It's a long, long road – it can be fine one day and terrible the next. You just have to keep believing that everybody has got the child's best interests at heart.

I'm very lucky, I came out of it and I've got a beautiful, six-year-old who is in relative good health. Yes, he's got his difficulties, but if they'd told me then what the problems would be, I would have taken it in a heartbeat."

Claudia, mum to Chase

Long-term issues

Extremely premature babies have a higher risk of developing behavioural and/ or health problems than babies born closer to term. However, there are lots of accessible treatments that can help your child as he grows.

Being born early can make babies vulnerable to a number of problems as they develop and grow up. The earlier a baby is born, the more likely he is to be diagnosed with a problem or condition. While most premature babies will be completely healthy as they get older, a few are likely to have at least some repercussions of their early birth, even if these are short-term. There are, however, various treatments and therapies available to help your baby develop and reach his full potential.

Respiratory problems Many premature babies, particularly those born before 30 weeks' gestation, suffer from longer-term respiratory problems. These can be partly because of the breathing difficulties commonly seen in premature babies, known as respiratory distress syndrome (RDS), which is due to their lungs being too immature to work properly. The earlier a baby is born, the more likely he is to develop RDS.

Babies can also have respiratory problems as a result of necessary interventions, such as ventilation, to help them breathe. These are life-saving treatments, but they cause pressure in the lungs, which carries the risk of damaging them. Babies who are still dependent on oxygen by the corrected gestational age of 36 weeks are said to have chronic lung disease of prematurity (see p.78). Over time the lungs usually grow and heal and most children are symptom-free by the age of two.

Babies with chronic lung disease are more likely to develop a cough and wheezing due to narrowed airways, resulting in episodes of breathing difficulty.

If your child does develop breathing problems, your doctor can prescribe inhalers to prevent or relieve symptoms. Attaching the inhaler to a "spacer" (see photo, opposite) makes it easier for children to use.

Infections Premature babies are more susceptible to infections, both while they are on the neonatal unit and for the first few months after coming home. They are at greater risk of contracting minor infections such as colds and other viral infections, and they are also more likely to be susceptible to major infections such as pneumonia and meningitis. Infections such as bronchiolitis (see p.107), which are often minor in an older, term baby can be devastating in a premature baby, particularly if he has other problems such as chronic lung disease.

Flattened heads Some premature babies have asymmetrical head shapes. This is normal and is usually a result of the baby lying more on one side than the other, causing his soft immature skull to flatten on this side. In many cases, the baby's head shape becomes more normal as he grows, but sometimes it persists or becomes worse.

You may see that your baby prefers to breastfeed on one side rather than the other, has restricted movements on one side, or has a preference to turn his head to one side. This is the result of a problem with his neck. A physiotherapist or an osteopath can improve the movement of the neck, and if it's done early enough, this can improve the capacity for normal, even growth of the head.

Cerebral palsy Cerebral palsy (CP) is a term that describes disorders of movement, coordination, and posture that are caused by a permanent injury to the brain. CP is not uncommon in significantly premature babies, and babies born earlier are at a higher risk. The injured brain is unable to send signals to coordinate the muscles and make them move. This results in tight, stiff muscles, causing difficulties in balancing, walking, and maintaining posture. There may also be problems with controlling facial movements and speech. As well as motor problems, some children with CP may have associated difficulties with sight, hearing, learning, and behaviour. They are also more likely to have epilepsy. Symptoms vary from severe to very mild, so doctors will watch your child closely to see how much he is affected.

There is no cure for CP, but there is a range of therapies available to treat all levels of the disorder. Physiotherapy may be started while a baby is on the neonatal unit, and continued when he goes home in order to encourage good positioning and prevent stiffening of his limbs. It may then continue throughout childhood at home, nursery, and school. Speech and language therapy may also be provided if your child is having difficulties in speech development. Medication may be prescribed to aid muscle movement, and, in some cases, surgery can help correct a lack of muscle function.

Behavioural problems Issues around behaviour are common in children who were born very prematurely. Sometimes these problems can be behavioural responses to difficulties with movement – often there is a pattern of muscular tension and restriction of the joints, which can exacerbate behavioural problems.

Premature babies may also be more likely to have attention deficit hyperactivity disorder (ADHD), which can cause inattention, restlessness, and

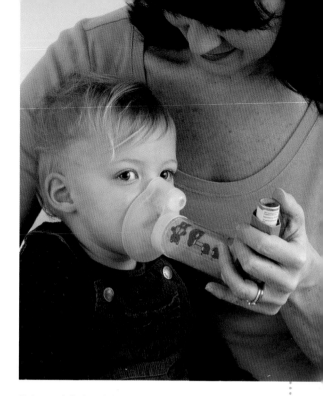

Using an inhaler Children born early are more likely to develop breathing problems. Make sure that anyone who cares for your child knows how to use his inhaler.

impulsive behaviour. They are also at greater risk of autistic spectrum disorders, which affect interaction, communication, and imagination, and can have a significant effect on their behaviour.

Learning difficulties Research has shown that being born very early may sometimes affect a child's ability to process information, which may be linked to learning difficulties, such as slower language development and problems with communication. Difficulties with motor skills can affect a child's ability to perform certain tasks, and behavioural problems such as inattention, impulsivity, and anxiety may also affect a child's ability to learn.

Children with learning difficulties may need extra support at school or it may be necessary for them to attend a special needs school.

Living with disability

It is distressing to learn that your child may be disabled. However, there are therapies available that can help with movement and speech problems, as well as practical skills, to enable her to reach her full potential.

Hearing that your baby is likely to be disabled is usually devastating. In the first few months, it is often difficult to predict the extent of the problems she is likely to have, and frustrating to hear that doctors won't be sure about important concerns you may have, such as whether she will ever learn to walk or talk, until she is several years old.

Sadly, if your baby does not reach the expected milestones and starts to fall behind, it becomes increasingly likely that she will have a disability. If you are told that this is likely, you will want to do everything you can to help your baby achieve her

Reaching milestones When a child is known to have significant disabilities, every little step in his development is an exciting milestone which the whole family can celebrate.

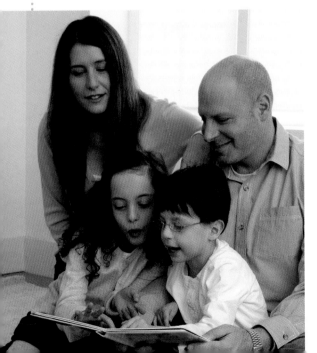

milestones. The therapists described below can help by showing you exercises to do with your baby. These are aimed at improving things such as muscle strength, stability, and speech, which in turn will help your baby to pick up new skills, and she may eventually catch up as she gets older and stronger. Certain disabilities, however, will need to be treated for the foreseeable future.

Occupational therapy Occupational therapists are usually trained in developmental care so they can help you to get familiar with your baby's behavioural cues. On the unit, they may spend time with your baby if she is irritable or having difficulties learning how to soothe herself.

Premature babies can easily become overloaded or over-stimulated and some are also sensitive to particular types of noise, light, or touch. Learning to observe your baby's behavioural cues can help you to see what her likes and dislikes are, and this will enable you to identify how much play and stimulation is right for your baby.

If necessary, an occupational therapist will advise you on what equipment you may need at home, for example in terms of seating, and on how your home may need to be adjusted according to your baby's specific needs. He or she may give you a programme to help your baby's development in terms of play and her fine motor skills.

Occupational therapy may become increasingly important in children with disabilities as they grow. It will help them gain skills in carrying out daily activities, such as eating, playing, and writing.

Physiotherapy Physiotherapists can offer guidance about positioning and handling your baby. They work closely with occupational therapists. They can advise you on how to position your baby if she has some head flattening due to her prematurity, and they will recommend activities to help correct it.

Therapists will give you advice about appropriate activities for your baby to help her develop her physical skills. For example, they'll recommend that your baby should have supervised awake '"tummy time" for a few minutes several times a day to help develop the skills needed later for crawling and to prevent head flattening. They will advise you that young babies should not spend long periods in car seats or baby bouncer seats as they need the freedom to kick around on a baby mat on the floor to help develop their muscle tone. Baby walkers (the kind with a seat in a wheeled frame) should be avoided as they encourage poor posture and can delay walking. They also enable babies to reach potential hazards.

Your child may need physiotherapy throughout her childhood, as it will give her the skills and abilities to become more independent and will greatly improve her quality of life.

Osteopathy This is concerned with movement of the body, and the underlying theory is that a body that moves well is able to work well. Osteopaths find that children born prematurely have different patterns of movement to term babies, and sometimes these unusual movements affect the child's health and development.

As they grow and develop, children who were born prematurely may face different problems that can sometimes be more frequent or greater than children who were born at term. Lots of families find that osteopathy can be a useful intervention for some of these issues, although so far there has been little formal research into this.

MY STORY

Dana says...

"When Max was in the unit, he had a massive bleed on the brain. The staff weren't sure if he was going to survive. He did survive, and the doctors knew he was brain damaged.

They told me he'd most likely have cerebral palsy, but they didn't know to what extent. They said he could be in a wheelchair for the rest of his life, not being able to feed himself, not being able to talk or breathe for himself... or he could be really bad at maths, or not be able to concentrate very well. I thought okay, so somewhere in between.

It was difficult for him to hold his head up as he had a very heavy head, so he never crawled but he eventually started sitting very, very late. Everything has been very late. Then he started progressing: he sat up and he eventually started moving around a little bit, bottom shuffling. Now he can walk holding my hand. He can walk beautifully. He talks but not very well, so he has speech therapy, physiotherapy, and occupational therapy, but he's in a mainstream school – he's just started in reception. He's clever, he's quite bright, but he's definitely behind, there's no doubt about it. With walking he's a couple of years behind but with everything else he's kind of catching up. And he's very good at maths! I can't tell you how amazed and how proud I am of him – he's just amazing, in every which way. **"**

Dana, mum to Erin and Max

Speech and language therapy This is mainly offered to babies who have difficulties in feeding. It assesses sucking and swallowing, and makes sure these are safe and that milk is not likely to spill into the lungs. As babies grow, they may have speech delay, and a speech and language therapist can advise parents how to help their child.

Your child's prognosis

It's natural for parents to want to know what their child's future prospects are, but it is often very hard to predict. In general, the more premature a baby was, the more likely he is to have problems, but each child is an individual.

Doctors will aim to be as honest as possible about your baby's prognosis. They can look at research showing that the percentage of babies with a certain type of scan will have long-term problems, but it is difficult to predict the full extent of these problems.

There is research that shows the likelihood of babies of each gestational age surviving and of having long-term problems. There are also data

old health professionals will refer to his CGA as "term plus two weeks". This means that allowances are made for the prematurity and your baby is not expected to be behaving like a 12-week-old baby but more like a two-week-old baby. In reality, if he is making good progress, he will be behaving more like a four-week-old baby – in other words he will be beginning to catch up.

> "She was the smallest on the ward and that was worrying. Now she's on the 90th percentile! She's absolutely fine – very funny, bright, and aware."
>
> *Carolyn, mum to Evie*

showing the likelihood of long-term problems in a baby who has been deprived of oxygen before or during birth. The extra knowledge gained from scans can be very helpful, but every baby is an individual and there are so many factors that can affect their development that parents, frustratingly, usually have to be patient.

In general, the earlier your baby was born and the sicker he was, the more likely he is to have long-term problems. The vast majority of babies born after 28 weeks' gestation will survive and have no major long-term problems. However, babies born at less than 25 weeks will survive and they will have significant problems.

For the first year or so, doctors usually refer to your baby's corrected gestational age (CGA). This is his actual age adjusted for prematurity. So if your baby was born 10 weeks early, when he is 12 weeks

Doctors and nurses also use the CGA to plot babies' growth on a chart. Many babies who have had a difficult time on the unit will grow very slowly initially and will need careful monitoring and advice on optimal nutrition. This is important not only for your baby's physical growth but also for his brain growth and therefore for long-term development.

It is likely that babies will have catch-up growth eventually and hopefully most premature and small-for-dates babies will reach their full genetic height potential.

Growth charts The charts opposite, based on growth charts published by the WHO, show expected growth for breastfed babies; bottle-fed babies gain weight slightly faster. The chart uses curves called centiles; 96 per cent of children who are developing normally will fall between the 2nd and 98th centiles. There are separate charts for boys and girls as boys are slightly heavier at a given age than girls.

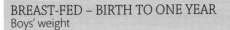

BREAST-FED – BIRTH TO ONE YEAR
Boys' weight

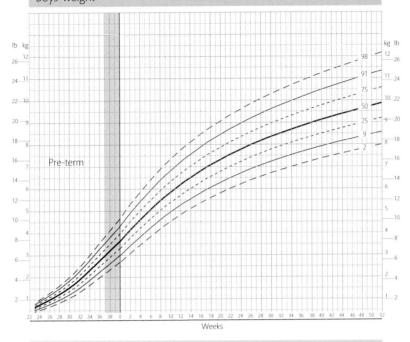

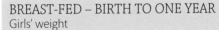

BREAST-FED – BIRTH TO ONE YEAR
Girls' weight

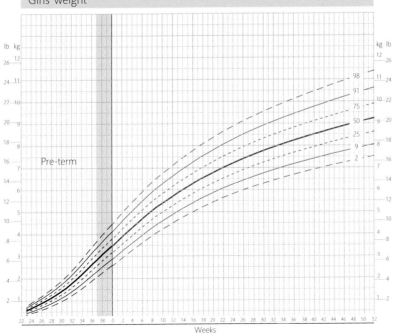

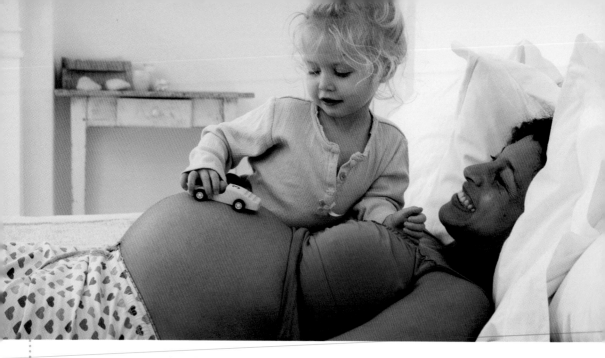

As your child grows

As you look back on the early weeks and months of your child's life, you'll realize how far you have come as a family. Whether or not your child has ongoing difficulties, you can now look to the future together.

The most important part of parenting a child who has been on a neonatal unit is to give her your love, time, and attention. For some parents it may be hard to bond with their baby initially, and you may feel you have a lot of lost time to make up. It's impossible to love a child too much, and spending time with her when you finally get home – talking to her, playing with her, and cuddling her – will all help her to feel secure and develop to her full potential

.

Your child's development If your child is experiencing any developmental or behavioural difficulties, she may be offered a place in a pre-school group that will meet her specific needs.

In time, if she needs a school for children with learning difficulties, your health care and local education teams will let you know what is available and what to do. Many children with more minor difficulties are able to go to mainstream school with support. If your child goes to a school for children with learning difficulties, all the therapists she needs will be on hand.

Your family life The more time you can spend with your child, both on your own and with friends and family, the more she will be able to develop as an individual and flourish.

Your child will not suffer if both of you are working as long as she is cared for by someone she

A special bond Once you're past the uncertainty of the early days, you may feel you have to make up for lost time. You may also be considering another pregnancy.

is close to. She will also benefit from interaction with other children in a nursery setting, so if you are a stay-at-home parent, try to find some local drop-in groups. This will be fun for your child and a great way for you to meet other parents in your area.

As well as making time for your child, it's important to make time for yourself and your relationship. Find a reliable babysitter who can cope with any problems your child may have and who your child feels secure with so you feel confident and can relax when you go out.

It's important to try to enjoy your family life as it is now and, if you can, avoid thinking about what developmental problems your child may have in the future, as this can be very daunting. Instead, focus on living in the moment.

What about your next pregnancy?

When you're thinking about having another child, it is natural for you to be worried that the baby will also be premature and you may have to relive the neonatal unit experience. If there was a clear reason for your pre-term labour, such as high blood pressure or placental abruption (where the placenta comes away from the wall of the womb), your obstetrician will discuss with you whether it is likely to happen next time and what can be done to prevent it. If there was no obvious reason, it is very likely that the next pregnancy will go to term.

However, that won't stop you worrying and you may well be offered more regular consultant-led follow-up. Even if you didn't see a consultant while you were pregnant, there will have been one responsible for you. So if you have any queries, ask your midwife or GP if you can see the consultant before planning your next pregnancy.

MY STORY

Dana says...

"**Erin is absolutely fine. She did have what they called chronic lung disease but she's fine now.**

When she was younger, until about four or five, when she had a cold, it lasted a long time. She'd be coughing for a month after a cold, just because her lungs were a little bit weak from being on the ventilator and oxygen for so long. She's grown out of that, and there's not one thing about her that you could see that shows she was premature.

She's very, very well. She's the same height as, even taller than, most of the girls in her class. She's very bright, too – she was speaking at one. She did everything early on, apart from physically. Physically it took her a long time. **"**

Dana, mum to Erin and Max

Growing and learning Playing with your child will be fun for both of you and will make her feel secure. The time you spend together will help her develop and flourish.

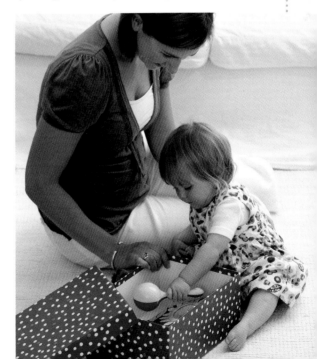

Meet the families

The parents quoted throughout this book all had babies who were cared for in the Starlight Neonatal Unit at Barnet Hospital, and they have shared their stories in the hope that they will help other parents in similar situations.

When we were writing this book, we were lucky enough to meet several families who were willing to talk openly about their experiences of prematurity and neonatal care.

Some of the babies in this book spent time at more than one hospital, so the comments from their mums and dads relate to a number of different neonatal units.

Wherever you are and whichever hospital your baby is in, the equipment, monitoring, treatment, and broad principles of care will be similar. The way each individual neonatal unit is run and the community support structure may vary from place to place, but the dedicated medical expertise and the emotional intensity for parents is the same all over the world.

Some names have been changed.

Chase, his mum Claudia and dad Daniel

Chase, now six, was born at 23 weeks and five days. Sadly, his identical twin brother, Alfie, was stillborn.

When Chase was born his parents were told he had a one per cent chance of survival. He was in hospital for seven and a half months and is now doing well, despite having some developmental challenges, which include global delay and autism.

Claudia says: "When I look at my son, what I see is a wonderful, unique child who has brought me an enormous amount of aggravation, but an enormous amount of love and joy. It's exceptionally challenging, but it's taught me a depth of love that I had no idea existed."

Erin and Max, their mum Dana and dad Peter

Erin, now eight, was born at 26 weeks. Her brother, Max, now five, was born at 25 weeks.

Erin weighed just 670g (1lb 8oz) when she was born. She improved quickly, and went home before her due date. Luckily she didn't develop any serious problems and she's fine now. Max struggles physically because he has cerebral palsy and can't use his right side very well. He has had an operation to insert a shunt to drain excess fluid from his brain and is making excellent progress.

Dana says: "A lot of people have said to me, it must be really hard what you've been through, you poor thing. I don't want anyone to feel sorry for me because I've got the most beautiful son, the most gorgeous, amazing child. And his sister is amazing, too – she's everything to him; they get on so well."

Freddie, his mum Jenni and dad Ross

Freddie was born at 28 weeks. Ross and Jenni knew that he was going to arrive early but when he was born weighing just 730g (1lb 9oz) they didn't yet know that he would be fighting for his life for months. Freddie has had to have a hernia operation, but is now thriving at home. Ross coped with the stress of Freddie's early weeks by starting a blog, which has more than 50,000 followers.

Ross says: "The day we brought Freddie home was magic – it was on his due date. It was an amazing feeling taking him home, the best day by far."

You can read all about Freddie's journey at freddiemcgill.blogspot.com

Jaden, his mum Kamini and dad Harish

Jaden was born at 27 weeks and spent 10 weeks in neonatal care. He has an older brother, Kamran, nearly three. Kamran and Jaden's brother, Shaant, was born at 23 weeks and sadly died shortly afterwards. Jaden left hospital soon after the time of writing and is thriving happily at home.

Kamini says: "We will never forget our baby Shaant that we lost, and I don't think that a day goes by that my husband and I do not think of him. I'm glad that we did not give up trying as we would never have had our two lovely boys Kamran and Jaden."

Evie, her mum Carolyn and dad Adam

Evie was born at 31 weeks. She has an older brother, Dexter, who is six.

After Evie's premature birth, Carolyn developed severe postnatal depression. Although it was a very difficult time, Carolyn managed to get the support and treatment she needed, and Evie is flourishing.

Carolyn says: "Evie is absolutely fine – very funny, bright, and aware. I'd really struggle to have any complaints at all about the way we were treated on the unit and the way we were looked after. They were all just marvellous."

Leo, his mum Shell and dad Bal
Leo was born at 23 weeks and three days. When Shell's waters broke unexpectedly early, hospital staff fought hard to save Leo. After many ups and downs, he was well enough to go home not long after Bal shared his experiences for this book.

Bal says: "The premature world brings out the best in people; it's one of the worst things that can happen in people's lives but it brings out the best in them. My dad said to me, 'Treat your son like a flower. It's your flower, you look after it and enjoy its scent and the way it looks and don't worry about anyone else's flowers.' And that's stuck with me. If people say commiserations – sorry to hear about your baby, you think, why are you saying sorry? My baby's alive!"

Samuel and Leo, their mum Sophie and dad Carlos
Twins Samuel and Leo were born at 26 weeks. Samuel did very well from the beginning, but Leo had lots of problems, struggling with many infections. Samuel went home three weeks before his due date, and Sophie and Carlos were able to take Leo home not long afterwards.

Sophie says: "I can remember clear distinctive moments when I bonded with them in the hospital. The first time I cleaned Samuel's face he was just looking straight at me. I remember it so clearly – it was: Bam! Instant! Wow! I couldn't cuddle Leo until later because he was so unwell, but I can feel the bonding happening now. I'm getting those little moments with him."

Xavier, his mum Cher and dad Nick
Xavier, now four, was born at 31 weeks. He has an older brother, Samuel, 10. Xavier was born prematurely because he had a heart condition called supraventricular tachycardia (SVT). After some scary ups and downs in the early days, Xavier is healthy and doing very well.

Cher says: "While Xav was in hospital I would always spend time holding his head and feet for comfort so he would know I was there. To this day, if he is lying near me he asks me to hold his feet or puts his foot on my leg. It's such a comfort to know that even when I couldn't hold him all the time I was still reassuring him and bonding with him."

Nick says: "All I wanted to know to begin with was, 'Will he be okay?' The consultants and nurses would talk medically about his condition, but nothing was sinking in, I just wanted to know if everything was going to be okay."

Glossary

When your baby is on the neonatal unit you'll hear lots of terms that may be unfamiliar. If there's anything you can't find in this glossary or you need further explanation, the staff on the unit should be happy to help.

Anaemia
A condition in which there is a low level of haemoglobin (the substance needed to carry oxygen) in the blood.

Apnoea
A period during which the baby stops breathing.

Blood gas
A test done on a sample of blood to assess the levels of oxygen, carbon dioxide, and acidity in the blood.

Bradycardia
A heart rate that is too slow.

Cerebral function monitor (CFM)
A device used to monitor the brain activity of a baby who is thought to be having seizures.

Cerebrospinal fluid (CSF)
The clear colourless fluid that bathes the brain and spinal cord. A tiny sample of this is sometimes taken for testing via a *lumbar puncture* if *meningitis* is suspected.

Continuous positive airways pressure (CPAP)
A method of providing support for a baby's breathing by blowing air or oxygen at increased pressure into the lungs through the nose. This stops the lungs from collapsing and makes it easier for the baby to breathe.

Congenital
From birth; a congenital condition is one that a baby is born with.

Corrected gestational age (CGA)
The actual age of a baby adjusted for prematurity. If your baby was born 10 weeks early, when he is 12 weeks old his corrected gestational age would be "term plus two weeks".

Cranial ultrasound
An ultrasound scan of the baby's brain through the soft spot on the head, called the *fontanelle*.

Desaturation
A significant decrease in the baby's oxygen level.

Echo or echocardiogram
An ultrasound scan of the heart.

Endotracheal (ET) tube
A plastic tube inserted into the baby's trachea (windpipe) via the mouth or nose and attached to a ventilator.

Enteral feeds
Feeds that go into the stomach, via a tube inserted through the nose (nasogastric) or the mouth (orogastric), if the baby is unable to suck.

Fontanelle
The soft spot on top of a baby's head, which closes at about one year of age.

Haemorrhage
Leakage of blood from veins or arteries into surrounding tissues.

Heart murmur
A noise caused by the flow of blood within the heart or through a blood vessel, which can be heard with a stethoscope. Heart murmurs are often found to be "innocent", meaning they are not caused by a structural problem within the heart. In premature babies, a murmur is often due to the sound of blood flowing through a *patent ductus arteriosis (PDA)*. A cardiac *echo* is usually used to decide whether the murmur is anything to worry about.

Hyaline membrane disease
A condition in which lack of *surfactant* in the baby's lungs leads to increased surface tension in the fluid lining the air sacs. This means it is harder for the baby to breathe in and overcome the forces holding the lung closed.

Hydrocephalus
An abnormal build-up of fluid within the skull, sometimes called "water on the brain"'. Hydrocephalus occurs when the flow of *cerebrospinal fluid (CSF)* around the brain and into the spinal cord is blocked, resulting in enlargement of the brain's ventricles (cavities where CSF is produced). If severe, and putting pressure on the brain, it may require surgical treatment.

Hypoglycaemia
Low blood sugar.

Hypoxic ischaemic encephalopathy (HIE)
Brain damage that can occur when the baby's brain is deprived of oxygen before or during the birth. It can be mild, moderate, or severe. If it's severe, your baby may be treated with cooling therapy to slow down the metabolism of the brain, which may restrict damage. In mild cases, the damage is usually temporary, but in severe cases, it's more likely to be permanent.

Intravenous fluids
Fluids infused into a baby's vein to provide water, sugar, and usually also salt and potassium.

Intraventricular haemorrhage (IVH)
A leakage of blood into the ventricles (fluid-filled cavities) in the brain.

Intra-uterine growth retardation (IUGR)
Sometimes also called "small for dates", a problem in which the baby fails to grow at the expected rate in the womb, so is born weighing too little.

Intubation
The procedure of placing an *endotracheal (ET) tube* into the baby's trachea (windpipe) to help him breathe. In an emergency it is done with no sedation for the baby, but if there is time the baby is sedated.

Jaundice
The yellow colour noticed in the eyes and skin due to an increased level of bilirubin (a substance produced when the liver breaks down red blood cells)

in the blood. It is common in term and premature babies.

Long line
A long, very thin and flexible silastic (silicone rubber) tube, which is skilfully inserted into a vein and fed along the vein almost as far as the heart. It is used to give *total parenteral nutrition (TPN)*.

Lumbar puncture (LP)
A method of obtaining a small quantity of *cerebrospinal fluid (CSF)* to check for *meningitis*. In the neonatal unit, LPs are often done on babies who have a raised temperature or seem unwell because it is difficult to rule out meningitis. An LP is sometimes also used to remove extra CSF if there is *hydrocephalus*.

Meconium
The baby's first poo, which is sticky and black.

Meningitis
A serious infection of the meninges, the layers of tissue covering the brain.

Necrotizing enterocolitis (NEC)
A very serious illness that affects some premature babies in which the gut becomes inflamed and ulcerated and can perforate.

Nitric oxide
A gas that is used as treatment for babies with certain problems, such as failure of the blood to circulate through the lungs.

Oedema
Swelling of a part of the body due to excess fluid leaking out of blood vessels.

Patent ductus arteriosis (PDA)
Before a baby is born, blood bypasses the lungs through a tiny blood vessel that connects the two large arteries that leave the heart: the aorta and the pulmonary artery. This hole, called the ductus arteriosis, has to close at birth so that blood can circulate through the lungs and pick up oxygen. In premature babies, it often stays open for a while and is known as a patent ductus arteriosis. If it causes problems in the baby, it may need to be closed by using a drug or by a small operation.

Pneumothorax
Literally "air in the chest". This happens when air leaks from a lung into the space between the lung and the ribcage. In severe cases, the lung collapses, and a chest tube has to be inserted to allow it to re-expand. Minor cases may not need treatment. It's more common in babies who need *ventilation* or *continuous positive airways pressure (CPAP)* to help with their breathing, but it sometimes occurs in babies who need no help.

Pulmonary haemorrhage
Leakage of blood into the lungs. It can be severe and is often life-threatening.

Retinopathy of prematurity (ROP)
Disorganized growth of blood vessels in the eye. In severe cases, it can lead to retinal detachment and blindness, and early detection is vital so that laser treatment can be offered to prevent progression of the disease. All very premature babies are at risk of ROP.

Respiratory distress syndrome (RDS)
A condition affecting the lungs of premature babies that results in rapid

breathing and low oxygen levels in the blood. The most common cause is lack of **surfactant**. However, it can also be caused by pneumonia (an infection of the lung), and for this reason, all babies with RDS are given antibiotics.

Sepsis
Another word for infection.

Septicaemia
Infection in the blood.

Surfactant
A substance produced in the lungs of unborn babies as they approach term. If they are born early, a lack of surfactant results in *hyaline membrane disease*. Surfactant is now produced artificially and given to premature babies via an *endotracheal (ET) tube* soon after birth. This greatly improves the baby's lungs and makes the baby easier to ventilate.

Tachycardia
A heart rate that is too fast.

Total parenteral nutrition (TPN)
Special fluids given to sick and premature babies who are unable to have milk feeds. It is given directly into a vein, and consists of protein, carbohydrate, salts, and fat.

Umbilical artery/vein catheter (UAC/UVC)
A long flexible silastic (silicone rubber) tube inserted into an umbilical artery or vein. A UAC is used to take blood samples and can also be used to monitor the baby's blood pressure. A UVC is used to give fluids and drugs.

Ventilation
The use of a machine called a ventilator to take over the work of breathing in babies who are too premature or too sick to breathe for themselves. Air is delivered directly into the baby's lungs via an *endotracheal (ET) tube*.

Resources

BLISS
Support for families of premature and special-care babies
www.bliss.org.uk
Helpline: 0500 618 140

Child Bereavement Charity
www.childbereavement.org.uk
Support and information:
01494 568900

Contact a Family
Support for families with disabled children
www.cafamily.org.uk
Helpline: 0808 808 3555

Cry-sis
Support for parents dealing with excessive crying
www.cry-sis.org.uk
Helpline: 08451 228669

Down's Syndrome Association
www.downs-syndrome.org.uk
Helpline: 020 8614 5100

Epilepsy Action
www.epilepsy.org.uk
Helpline: 0808 800 5050

FSID (Foundation for the Study of Infant Deaths)
fsid.org.uk
Helpline: 0808 802 6868

Hyperactive Children's Support Group
www.hacsg.org.uk
Tel: 01243 539966

La Leche League
Mother-to-mother support for breastfeeding
www.laleche.org.uk
Helpline: 0845 120 2918

Meningitis Trust
www.meningitis-trust.org
Helpline: 0808 801 0388

The National Autistic Society
www.autism.org.uk
Helpline: 0808 800 4104

Scope
Information on cerebral palsy
www.scope.org.uk
Helpline: 0808 800 3333

TAMBA (Twins and Multiple Birth Association)
www.tamba.org.uk
Twinline: 0800 138 0509

Tommy's
Research on stillbirth, premature birth, and miscarriage
www.tommy's.org

Index

Acknowledgments

Authors' acknowledgments

A huge thank you to **Sally Watkin**, who carried out all the interviews with parents and read through endless drafts.

Thanks to our editors **Andrea Bagg** and **Lizzie Yeates** for their skill and patience, and **Vanessa Davies** for taking wonderful photos. Thanks also to **Peggy Vance**, **Saskia Janssen**, **Dawn Henderson**, **Anne Fisher**, and the DK team.

We are grateful to **Dr Jane Hawdon** and **Andy Cole** from Bliss for their valuable comments.

We would also like to thank the following people for their invaluable contributions: **Cher Johnston,** specialist paediatric liaison nurse (psychology services); **Jo Wong**, matron, Starlight Neonatal Unit; **Karina Wyles**, neonatal clinical facilitator/community nurse specialist; **Margaret Jacobs**, housekeeper, Starlight Neonatal Unit; **Bernadette Henderson**, senior physiotherapist; **Panchali Shah**, physiotherapist; **Betty Hutcheon**, senior occupational therapist; **Andrew Maddick**, osteopath; **Mandy Lovett**, baby massage expert; **Silvia Konig**, neonatologist; and all the other staff on the Starlight Neonatal Unit, along with other expert friends and colleagues, who have given their time and expertise during the writing, editing, and photography.

Thank you too to all the families who have shared their experiences. We couldn't have done it without you!

Publisher's acknowledgments

DK would like to thank the parents of all the babies who appear in this book for allowing us to photograph them and their babies, and for their kind permission to reproduce their photographs.

Thank you to **Claire Cross** for proofreading, **Marie Lorimer** for the index, and **Charlotte Johnson** for picture research.

Picture credits

The publisher would also like to thank the following for their kind permission to reproduce their photographs:

(Key: a-above; b-below/bottom; c-centre; f-far; l-left; r-right; t-top)

1 Getty Images: Science Photo Library (c). **2 Science Photo Library:** Mark Thomas (c). **7 Science Photo Library:** John Thys / Reporters (c). **16 Getty Images:** Science Photo Library (bl). **22 Corbis:** commentsBernd Vogel (c). **24 Getty Images:** Science Photo Library (cb). **26 Getty Images:** ERproductions Ltd (ca). **30 Science Photo Library:** Penny Tweedie (bl). **39 Corbis:** Philippe Lissac / GODONG/ Godong (r). **46 Alamy Images:** Science Photo Library (c). **48 Getty Images:** Science Photo Library (ca). **54 Science Photo Library:** AJ Photo (bl). **74 Science Photo Library:** AJ Photo (cb). **84 Corbis:** Ruth Jenkinson / Science Photo Library (c). **87 Science Photo Library:** Mark Thomas (fbr). **110 Mother & Baby Picture Library:** Ian Hooton (cra)

Growth charts: adapted from charts provided by the Child Growth Foundation, London

Jacket images: *Front:* Dreamstime.com: Vividpixels (c); Getty Images: Science Photo Library (cl); *Back:* **Alamy Images:** Science Photo Library (tr); **Getty Images:** ERproductions Ltd (tl); Science Photo Library (ftl); *Spine:* Dreamstime.com: Vividpixels

All other images © Dorling Kindersley
For further information see: **www.dkimages.com**